T0273300

A LIFETIME OF
SENSATIONAL
SMILES

A LIFETIME OF SENSATIONAL SMILES

TRANSFORMING LIVES THROUGH ORTHODONTICS

DR. KERRY WHITE BROWN

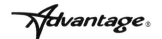

Published by Advantage, Charleston, South Carolina.
Member of Advantage Media Group.

ADVANTAGE is a registered trademark, and the Advantage colophon is a trademark of Advantage Media Group, Inc.

Printed in the United States of America.

10 9 8 7 6 5 4 3 2 1

ISBN: 978-1-59932-803-4
LCCN: 2017958325

Cover design by Melanie Cloth.
Layout design by George Stevens.

This publication is designed to provide accurate and authoritative information in regard to the subject matter covered. It is sold with the understanding that the publisher is not engaged in rendering legal, accounting, or other professional services. If legal advice or other expert assistance is required, the services of a competent professional person should be sought.

Advantage Media Group is proud to be a part of the Tree Neutral® program. Tree Neutral offsets the number of trees consumed in the production and printing of this book by taking proactive steps such as planting trees in direct proportion to the number of trees used to print books. To learn more about Tree Neutral, please visit **www.treeneutral.com.**

Advantage Media Group is a publisher of business, self-improvement, and professional development books. We help entrepreneurs, business leaders, and professionals share their Stories, Passion, and Knowledge to help others Learn & Grow. Do you have a manuscript or book idea that you would like us to consider for publishing? Please visit advantagefamily.com or call **1.866.775.1696.**

To Gregory, my husband, and Greg Anthony II and Kerrington, our two sons, who tolerated my having missed several games and movies as I spent time writing and editing this book. Thank you all for your patience and support, your understanding, and, most importantly, your love.

TABLE OF CONTENTS

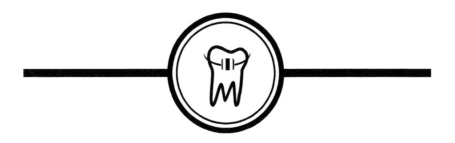

INTRODUCTION

I t's a question nearly every patient, adult or child, asks me at some point: "What made you decide to be an orthodontist?" They're always surprised when I tell them it started in third grade during Career Week. Our teacher asked us all what we wanted to be when we grew up and I said, "A dental hygienist!"

I admit it was an unusual response, but my dentist was an unusual guy. He always found a way to make visits to his office fun—in fact, I actually looked forward to them. Somehow, he was able to charm me out of being nervous or afraid, even when he needed to give me a shot. That intrigued me, and I decided I wanted to do that, too.

My teacher said, "You know that to become a dental hygienist you'd have to take a lot of math and science classes. So why not become a dentist?"

I considered that for a split second and said, "Okay." From that moment on I started my journey to become a dentist. I decided I wanted to do orthodontics around the twelfth grade. My dentist had told me I needed braces, but my parents couldn't afford them. I realized then I wanted to be able to fix peoples' smiles. My parents were not tremendously career oriented but they were supportive, and it helped that my older brother (I'm the youngest of eight children) went to dental school, though he ultimately decided it wasn't for him.

I've always set high standards for myself, nobody imposed that on me, and I wasn't happy if I wasn't at the top of my class. I graduated from high school as the class valedictorian. I attended Benedict College and graduated Summa Cum Laude with a Bachelor of Science in Chemistry. Then, I attended Howard University College of Dentistry in Washington, DC. The course work was rigorous, but my interest and determination didn't falter.

When I finished dental school, I went straight into orthodontic residency. It was eye opening, because you're looking at things differently: the teeth, the jaws, how they work together, plus the technology involved, getting used to bending wires to make the teeth move the way you want them to move. It was like starting over. Fortunately, I've always been a techie, and I still get excited about learning new technology and how I can use it to help my patients.

When I graduated, I went to work in orthodontics in a general dentist's office in my hometown, ultimately buying my first practice about two hours away, then opening another across town. Not long after this I bought a third practice, and then a fourth location a few years later.

Between having a growing family and a full-time workload, it's been a challenge—but I love a challenge, and having this kind of business allows me to do other things that are important to me, like charity work to help children who desperately need (but can't afford) orthodontics, which I find tremendously rewarding.

In working with our patients, we're very sensitive to their challenges; that's why we rotate our office hours to be accommodating. We open early and late on certain days because many of our adult patients need those times to fit in with their working schedules. As a working mom, I understand the challenges of fitting appointments into an already overstuffed agenda, and flexibility is much appreciated. To that end, we have even decided to offer Saturday hours in our practice. This decision definitely helps out those busy moms who can't fit another appointment in during their work-week.

In some ways, my agenda as a practitioner is still what it was when I was in third grade: to make the experience of going through treatment enjoyable and fun for all my patients, young or old, and to be the best possible orthodontist I can be.

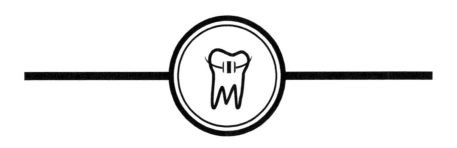

CHAPTER 1

WHAT IS AN ORTHODONTIST, AND WHY DO YOU NEED ONE?

I get that question more often than you might think, but since dentists and orthodontists alike all work on teeth, the differences aren't always as clear to a layperson (or to a new patient) as one might think.

I should start out by saying all orthodontists are dentists, but not all dentists are orthodontists. In dental school, the student will learn how to restore and replace missing teeth and parts of teeth that are damaged by decay or periodontal (gum) disease. We all begin there—but to become an orthodontist, you must enroll in an additional two to three years of specialty training. It's only after graduating from an accredited four-year dental school that you can apply for orthodontic residency programs. Some of these residency programs take two years to complete, however most of them now take three years to complete.

The orthodontist's scope is quite different from that of a general dentist. In lay terms, the general dentist is looking at the general health of the mouth, checking teeth to see if they're decayed and need filling, or whether you need a cleaning. For an orthodontist, the focus is, "Are the teeth and the jaws aligned properly? Do they work well together? Are there any muscular issues or skeletal problems that prevent the healthy function of the teeth and the jaws?" In an orthodontic residency, you learn how to diagnose, prevent, and intercept problems with the teeth and the jaws and how they come together, whether you're looking at a child's developing jaw or an adult jaw.

While some dentists do offer some orthodontic services, they are typically limited to a few less complex procedures. The thousands of extra hours we orthodontists spend learning the mechanics of tooth movement really pay off for our patients, because we're not only equipped to deal with much more complex cases, but we're also able to address relatively simple cases with a larger number of possible solutions. We can fine-tune those treatments and combine them to create the ideal solution for each patient's unique case. There's no one-size-fits-all solution, because every mouth is as unique as the person it belongs to, and I like to think that a good orthodontist combines an artist's eye with a clinician's expertise to make a patient's desired results a reality.

WHAT MIGHT BRING YOU TO AN ORTHODONTIST'S OFFICE?

Patients come to the orthodontic office because their general dentist or pediatric dentist has referred them to us, or they will self-refer. Your dentist may have told you that your child's teeth aren't coming in properly, or you could see for yourself they're not lining up as they should. Your dentist may tell you, "Your son isn't losing his teeth in a timely fashion and his permanent teeth are coming in, so things are getting pushed out of place." A dentist may be the first to notice that your bite isn't coming together properly and will refer you for a consultation with an orthodontist.

When I talk about "self-referred," I mean that in the case of some adults, they will look in a mirror and say, "I don't like the way my teeth look," or, "I don't like the way my bite comes together," and will subsequently call and set up a smile assessment appointment (consultation) for themselves. Often with adults they've been unhappy with their smiles for years, but for whatever reason they weren't able to get the work done before. Many people don't know that orthodontists do not require a reference from a general dentist before they'll see you for a smile assessment.

If you're the parent of a child with misaligned teeth, you may see that your child is suffering the social pangs that a less-than-sensational smile can cause. We see children in that situation quite often, because their peers can be cruel. There can be teasing and name-calling aimed at a child whose teeth stick out or are otherwise unsightly, and that can quickly become a self-esteem/social issue for that child. Parents bring their child in saying, "He's complaining that kids are picking on him," or, "She's complaining she has a gap between her front teeth and she doesn't like how it looks." I feel strongly that issues that are negatively impacting a child's self-image or social interactions must be addressed as early as possible, because the sooner they feel less self-conscious about how they look, the happier and more self-assured they'll be.

WHY DO YOU NEED AN ORTHODONTIST?

The most obvious issues—like protruding or misaligned teeth—are the easiest to spot, and are what most often brings those patients who self-refer to our practice. But, of course, there are many problems orthodontists can address that are harder to spot than these.

As an example, we had a fifteen-year-old in recently. Tom had a tooth that should have come in when he was seven or eight years old but that tooth had still not erupted, although all of his other permanent teeth were in. Of course, that primary (baby tooth) wasn't obvious to parents who said, "I don't see any spaces. All the teeth are there." Unfortunately, Tom's permanent tooth was still impacted (up in the bone).

Often, parents will bring a child in because the child has **problems chewing** and it's limiting their food choices. Parents may not know why their child doesn't like to eat one food or another, and sometimes that's unfairly written off to fussiness, when it might actually be because it hurts them to eat that particular food, or they can't chew it well. We attribute this to the occlusion, how their teeth come together. Jaws that shift, make sounds, and are painful, or protruding jaws or retruding jaws—these are things that can cause discomfort but which don't necessarily jump out at parents as a potential problem because, they tell us, "He looks just like his dad, so I didn't think it was a problem." An orthodontist has the training to spot and treat these issues.

Protruding teeth are easily spotted, but some children bite their cheeks and Mom might say, "Oh, simply slow down. You're eating too fast." Often, it's because of the occlusion. A bite so deep that the lower teeth are hitting the roof of the mouth is also a problem that would probably prevent a child from eating something that requires more chewing and grinding, and can cause them to reject certain foods as it's too difficult or painful to eat. Those are things that we as orthodontists can spot, issues that could be musculature and could be a result of how the teeth and the jaws come together.

Some people habitually **grind or clench their teeth**. Often this is because of a prematurity in how the teeth hit when they're closing their mouth. Sometimes the grinding occurs because they're steadily trying to find a comfortable bite, so they grind, or come up with other parafunctional habits that in the long run are not good for the joints, or for the teeth themselves.

Mouth breathing is another issue that an orthodontist might need to address, because it can indicate a constricted airway. If the patient has a very narrow arch and we expand it, we also expand the base of the nose; now the airway is more open and the child can breathe more easily. There are some other conditions that the orthodontist is often the first to notice. Sometimes with a constricted airway expansion is not enough. Referring the child to an Ear, Nose, and Throat (ENT) doctor for a tonsils-adenoid removal helps the child breathe better and reduces the mouth breathing tendency, which over time could affect the way the jaws come together and how the child will grow. When the mouth is always hanging down and open, instead of horizontal growth we'll see a more vertical growth pattern, because of the posture of the lower jaw. This usually results in an open bite (teeth not coming together), another discrepancy that must be corrected by the orthodontist.

Expanding the arch and bringing the lower jaw forward can sometimes solve issues with **snoring or sleep apnea**. When the tongue is not dropping back into the airway when the child sleeps, the child can breathe, so snoring goes away. They're going to have a better quality of life because they're resting better and getting deeper sleep rather than interrupted sleep. Poor sleep can affect a child in many ways—mood, activity level, how they do in school, and can even cause weight gain.

Did you know that **speech impediments** can sometimes be the result of problems with the teeth? Some patients we get are referred for just that reason. Perhaps they sucked their thumb as a child, so their bite doesn't close, or there's no overlapping of the upper and lower front teeth (open bite). Many patients with these kinds of issues also have speech impediments, such as lisps—there are certain sounds they can't form because their teeth don't overlap, which won't allow them to place their tongue properly.

As bad as it is for a child to have awful-looking teeth, imagine how much tougher it is for them socially if that's combined with a speech impediment. We see children who are in special speech instruction at school, or who come in tongue-tied, and the actual underlying medical issue has never been diagnosed. When we're performing our clinical exam, we'll say, "Lift your tongue," and if the child can't lift his tongue, we can be sure that he or she has a speech impediment. We refer those cases to a periodontist to get their frenum attachment clipped (a minor procedure called a frenectomy) so that the child's tongue will have freedom of motion, allowing for their speech impediment to improve dramatically or simply vanish with proper therapy.

We treat children who suffer from open bites with orthodontics so they get proper closure. Now they can speak like an ordinary person, without having to think about how to make a particular sound. Sometimes the speech therapist can see that there are obvious issues with the teeth and the bite and will ask the parent, "Have you thought about taking your child to the orthodontist?" Other times, the child's dentist will refer them to the orthodontist.

One of my adult patients, who had a really large open bite, suffered with a serious lisp her entire life. We put her in treatment, closed down her bite, and suddenly her lisp was gone. She couldn't believe it—talk about a life-changing transformation! She told me, "I feel like a new person!"

WHY DO PARENTS AVOID TAKING THEIR CHILD TO THE ORTHODONTIST?

There are a few factors that can affect a parent's decision about consulting an orthodontist for their child. One worry is that orthodontics is expensive, and I often meet with people who think it costs much more than it really does. In our practice, as in many others, doctors have worked out ways to make orthodontics more affordable for the average family by not requiring big down payments. And it's important to realize that orthodontics is an investment in your child's health and future.

Sometimes parents are concerned because they've heard braces are painful, and they worry whether their child will be able to tolerate that. Yes, there is going to be some discomfort, but as far as pain, what fearful parents have in their minds is nothing close to what the orthodontic patient actually experiences. Technology has improved tremendously, as have our materials; these allow us to apply much lighter force over a longer period of time than what once was the case. Braces generally are far less clunky and uncomfortable than they used to be, too. Within a week or so people easily adjust to wearing them, especially children, and if there is any initial discomfort, it can be easily managed with over-the-counter pain medication for the first few days if needed. As a doctor, my experience is that even the patients who were the most skittish and nervous to begin with get over that quickly and are pleasantly surprised by how easy the process is.

Adults are sometimes more fearful initially than children. A woman in her thirties came in for a smile assessment recently because she'd suffered with ugly, out-of-aligned teeth her whole life and had finally gotten to the point where she was willing to undergo whatever torture (as she imagined it to be) was necessary to give her the smile she'd always wanted. We talked her through every step of the process, calming her as we went along—and she was fine.

Often, I'm convinced the fear springs from a lack of information; patients don't really know what to expect, and, as a result, are expecting the worst. After it's all said and done, they realize, "Oh my goodness, I was nervous for no reason at all."

CAN I TELL IF MY CHILD WILL NEED BRACES BASED ON THE SPACING OF THEIR BABY TEETH?

Even if your child's baby teeth are perfect, this isn't necessarily an indication that his or her adult teeth will come in properly. If baby teeth are crowded, you can be sure that the adult teeth will have crowding issues.

Among the most common issues we see is what's called a **crossbite**, where the upper teeth sit behind the lower teeth like a bulldog's. You need to correct crossbite early because, when your child has crossbite, it can actually damage the supportive tissue around those lower front teeth that are hitting the upper teeth improperly. Every time they bite down, they're pushing against those lower-front teeth. Remember, these are permanent teeth now, so pushing those teeth forward is making the bone in front very thin. They're literally pushing the teeth out of the bone and destroying the supporting structures around the lower front teeth. What happens when you don't have support around the root of the tooth? Well, ultimately the tooth falls out.

Before we see destruction of tissue in a child with a crossbite we want to correct it so there's no problem for the child as he gets older. We don't want to leave this periodontal issue unaddressed for too long because this could lead to the need for grafting and gingival flap surgeries due to sustained damage to the lower supporting structures as a result of the way the child was biting.

Dentists often refer children with problems like these because they're the first ones to see the ongoing destruction of the supporting tissue and know that this must be addressed quickly.

We can also address bad habits before they do real damage. Thumb or tongue sucking habits can wreak havoc on alignment, and demands correcting. What can an orthodontist do to help break this habit? First and foremost, if the habit is still ongoing, we can have the child wear devices or habit appliances to stop them, and to stop further damage to the teeth and supporting structures. After appliance therapy, braces will correct problems that have already occurred due to the habit. Keep in mind that the sooner the habit is broken the better, because less damage is done.

HOW OLD DOES MY CHILD NEED TO BE TO VISIT AN ORTHODONTIST?

According to the American Association of Orthodontists, seven is the ideal age for a first visit to the orthodontist, because that's when a specialist can see whether teeth spacing is adequate or if the bite is off. Early treatment is the best option, because when the child's mouth is growing we can take advantage of the growth process. Corrective measures early on can save more extensive work down the line, so it's worth an assessment visit just to make sure that everything is coming in properly for so many reasons. Preventing surgeries later in life is one, because sometimes if there are impacted or permanent teeth that aren't coming in correctly we can perform interceptive treatment. This could be as simple as taking out some baby teeth to allow space for the permanent teeth to come in, or so the erupting permanent tooth will shift and come in at a more favorable position. If there is an impacted tooth, sometimes catching them early enough allows us to guide them back into their correct path. If it's too late, then the patient is referred to the oral surgeon to have that impacted tooth removed. This creates a whole cascade of related problems; now that you have other teeth that have shifted out of place, you're looking at orthodontics as well as an implant later. Consequently, early assessment and early intervention are vital to a child with potential dental problems. Most of the time these problems are first spotted upon assessment by the orthodontist.

The good news? Sometimes if you start children early enough you can prevent having to take out permanent teeth because you can start widening the arches and creating space for the erupting permanent teeth. Sometimes if we wait too long, space has been lost and can't be regained. Then, our only option is to remove permanent teeth—that are usually healthy—to correct a crooked bite. We (parents and clinicians alike) always want to avoid removing permanent teeth if at all possible.

When a child is young, biology is on our side if work needs to be done. The longer you wait, the longer and more complex treatment becomes. Why put it off?

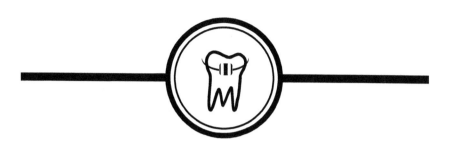

CHAPTER 2

WHAT A SENSATIONAL SMILE GIVES YOUR CHILD

O ne of the most gratifying things about my job is having the opportunity to give people their smiles back—and it's always rewarding. My first encounter with the impact that orthodontics can have was during my residency program. My patient in residency was an introverted twelve-year-old boy who had a really bad overbite. His front teeth just stuck out beyond his lip. He always walked with his head down. Any time I talked to him, he never raised his head or looked me in the eyes. At the time, not realizing how a person's smile could affect their self-esteem, I simply thought, "Okay, he's just a little shy."

About a year into his treatment his protrusion had corrected tremendously, and suddenly, he emerged from his shell; he talked all the time, and looked you right in the eye when you were talking to him. I could tell it wasn't just him outgrowing adolescent shyness, but it was more about feeling confident and comfortable with his smile and his overall appearance. He was a different child, and a much happier child. I remember thinking, *if braces can do that, then I'm all in.*

When you have ugly teeth, you learn very early in life not to show your smile because to smile is to draw attention to your looks, and that's the last thing you want. This habit of hiding your smile—whether it's covering your mouth when you laugh, turning away, or just not smiling at all—starts early and becomes second nature as one grows up. Often, people with "hidden" smiles become introverts when that may not really be their genuine character, and only when their teeth are fixed do their real, people-loving personalities show themselves.

Another instance of a big personality change I saw was in an adult patient whom I treated about two years ago. Mary works as a realtor, and because she's constantly talking to people, she wanted to feel more confident about the way her teeth looked. She wasn't looking for perfection, she told me, just for a better smile. She didn't want to go into traditional braces; she wanted to be treated with Invisalign because she didn't want the braces themselves to be a distraction when she was talking to her clients. We completed her Invisalign and Mary was ecstatic with the outcome. She felt far more confident in her ability to do business going forward because, for the first time, she felt good about the way she appeared to others.

Currently I'm working with Julie, a beautiful woman in her late-twenties who was so disheartened by her smile that she never showed her teeth. She was not confident at all. She told me during her smile assessment, "I never smile. I hate my smile. I hate talking to people because I don't like the way my teeth look."

I said to her, "You are gorgeous. What are you talking about? Your teeth are just a small part of your face." But to her it was everything.

We got her started in treatment about five months ago as of this writing. I can tell Julie's starting to feel better about her smile; it's already noticeably better, and her attitude is improving right along with it.

As I mentioned, children can be cruel to each other about appearance, and being the target of mockery or bullying leaves a real mark on a child's psyche. The pressure only gets worse as they get older. The stress of dealing with the kind of social ostracism that bad teeth can cause can make your child disappear. They're less likely to put themselves forward, to raise their hand in class, or to participate in activities—that holds them back from realizing their true potential, both in school and out.

Often the child will confide in me at that first assessment visit that he's having a hard time in school. It's usually later in treatment that you can tell they don't have that issue anymore, because you can see their personalities blossom and they actually talk more. I had a young patient of about fourteen whose grandmother brought her in. She's a beautiful young girl, but her teeth were pretty bad and she was mortified by how they looked. They were terribly crowded, almost stacked on top of each other. She'd fallen into the habit of keeping her lips closed when she smiled and dipping her head when she spoke; it was sad to see this clearly long-standing habit she'd developed out of self-consciousness and a lackluster smile. But, the last time I saw her at the clinic for her appointment, she'd found her smile—and a big, bright, beautiful smile it was, too. I said, "I remember how everything was when you got started."

She just beamed at me: "Oh, yes, I just love my teeth now."

You could tell that she definitely was much more self-assured in her appearance. She now spends an hour each morning on her make-up because she is so into how she looks with her new much-improved smile.

Sometimes malocclusions (when the teeth don't come together properly) can be hereditary, thus the parent has gone through a similar experience. I remember one parent who was in tears when she came in the first time because her child was being picked on and she had faced similar bullying in her youth about the appearance of her teeth. She didn't want her child to go through the pain she had suffered. It was very personal to her. She knew how it felt, and she told me, "I don't care what I need to do—I don't want my child to go through what I did."

A SMILE CAN CHANGE YOUR LIFE—LITERALLY!

And, of course, how you feel about yourself isn't just important when you're a child—how you saw yourself then and how you see yourself as an adult can impact your choices and options throughout your life. I recently read that scientists have determined that the human eye can judge a crooked smile in less than a second. Other research has suggested that people with attractive smiles do better in life—they're more social, have higher paying jobs, and report greater satisfaction and happiness in life.[1] We all know it's not fair to judge a book by its cover, but that's just what society does.

---

1   Christopher Ingraham, "Want People to Think You're Smarter? Smile More," *The Washington Post*, April 7, 2014, www.washingtonpost.com/news/wonk/wp/2014/04/07/

It's been shown that smiling has a positive physical effect on you, too; smiling more often can be very beneficial to your well-being, and can improve your mood and reduce stress. Penn State University did a study—the results of which were published in January 2005— in which they found that people who smile more tend to be seen as more likeable, more courteous and even more competent. It's not really surprising, as common sense tells us that if you smile, others are more likely to smile back at you, creating a happier environment. If everyone is smiling, that's more than likely not going to be an environment where people tend to be grumpy or disrespectful. It's going to be a much warmer environment. In fact, there's research from two studies done in 2002 and 2011 by scientists at Uppsala University in Sweden that concluded that frowning when looking at someone smiling is possible, but it's very difficult. Even a fake or a forced smile has a positive effect on your mood; it decreases your stress levels.[2]

Smiling lowers stress and anxiety by releasing endorphins, which are the chemicals in your body that make you happier. Smiling strengthens your immune system, and amazingly even helps your body produce white blood cells to help fight illnesses. In October 2011, Hungarian health research teams studying smiles published evidence that sick children who were made to smile increased their white blood cell count and increased the number of lymphocytes by 8.43 percent.[3]

A 2004 study by Penn State University showed that smiling makes you more approachable. In June 2012, University of Pittsburg published a study showing that smiling makes you seem trustworthy.

want-people-to-think-youre-smarter-smile-more/?utm_term=.387c111a9bbe

2   Vivian Giang, "How Smiling Changes Your Brain," *Fast Company*, January 30, 2015, www.fastcompany.com/3041438/how-smiling-changes-your-brain

3   A. Béres, Z. Lelovics, P. Antal, G. Hajós, A. Gézsi, A. Czéh, E. Lantos, and T. Major, "'Does Happiness Help Healing?' Immune Response of Hospitalized Children May Change during Visits of the Smiling Hospital Foundation's Artists," *Orvoi Hetilap*, 152(43): 1739-1744, www.ncbi.nlm.nih.gov/pubmed/21983400

Researchers at the University of Montpellier in France discovered that smiling is a more effective leadership technique than having great management ability. It all goes right back to smiles making you more likeable, because if people like you as a leader, then they are more apt to do what you ask of them.[4]

All in all, when you look at the research, a child that has a smile she's happy with makes her a healthier person overall. It allows people to see her in a more positive light, versus someone that's always frowning or not smiling at all. Buddhist monk Thich Nhat Hahn wrote, "Sometimes your joy is the source of your smile, but sometimes your smile can be the source of your joy."[5]

I remember the first time I really understood how important a good smile was. When I was in the first week of my residency program, the upperclassmen took all of the underclassmen out for lunch. When we all started talking, one of the upperclassmen jumped into the conversation and for the first time we all saw his teeth. Oh, my gosh—they looked awful, and were pointing in all directions. It immediately and completely changed the way we perceived him. Then, amazingly, he popped them out—it was a set of theatrical false teeth. We had a discussion about it afterward and he said, "What did you guys think about how I looked when I had those teeth in?"

This was the same upright guy in a button-down shirt that I had seen an hour prior—but he looked like a totally different person with those goofy teeth. I also assumed that his personal hygiene was bad, and that he wasn't someone that I would have wanted to approach and have a conversation with. That was a great exercise for us first-

---

4   Alyssa Detweier, "9 Surprising Reasons Why You Should Smile More," *Inspiyr.com*, 2014, http://inspiyr.com/9-benefits-of-smiling

5   Ronald Riggio, "There's Magic in Your Smile," *Psychology Today*, 2017, www.psychologytoday.com/blog/cutting-edge-leadership/201206/theres-magic-in-your-smile

year residents in how a person's smile really affects not only them, but also how other people see them.

IS MY CHILD MATURE ENOUGH TO BE RESPONSIBLE FOR HIS OR HER BRACES? CAN WE AFFORD THEM?

There are two big worries parents have when they're contemplating getting their child braces. Very often a parent will tell me, "I don't think my child's mature enough to care for braces," meaning they can't be trusted to keep their teeth clean and to not tear up the appliances. Will they follow the rules and—for instance—not eat a piece of taffy? Or will they just shrug and bite in? This has to do with the parent's assessment of their child's maturity level. Usually they're also thinking about their brushing habits—is their hygiene good enough that they can be trusted to care for their teeth and their braces while they're going through orthodontics?

The answer is, it depends on both of you. As the parent, you'll have to take on some oversight responsibility to make sure your child is taking proper care of their teeth. We can help, and will teach the child how to perform whatever additional steps are required to keep their teeth clean, but creating these new habits will require some collaboration with the parent to make sure the job is getting done. And, while children occasionally will mess up and bite into something they aren't supposed to, that usually happens only once, if at all.

Give your child the gift of a better future, because a good smile is going to outlast any other investment you can make on their behalf. Your child's smile just gains in value as they grow up. Just as you would do everything you could to help your child if there was some cosmetic deformity that marred their looks, you should also see that their smile can make a tremendous difference in the path they take as their calling card in life. Of course, we love our children—they look great to us, regardless of how their teeth look—but not everybody is going to see past that bad smile to the great person that's in there.

HOW DO YOU PUT A PRICE ON SELF CONFIDENCE?

So much of life depends on how big we dare to dream, and our self-confidence plays a large part in dictating the size of those dreams. British author James Allen said it well: "You are today where your thoughts have brought you. You will be tomorrow where your thoughts will take you." If today you're saying to yourself, "I'm not attractive, I'm not happy, I'm not confident," then how is that mindset going to get you to the CEO position at some top-notch Fortune 500 company? Or into medical school? If you're thinking, "I'm less than," or, "I'm not capable because I'm ashamed of what I look like," this mentality is not going get you there, because your mindset is not going to be, "I can reach for the stars."

Author Vic Johnson in his book *13 Secrets of World-Class Achievers* said, "Big doers are big dreamers." If we don't give our children what they need to be confident, then our children won't have what they need to dare to dream lofty dreams and accomplish their potential in life. In the classic Napoleon Hill book, *Think and Grow Rich,* Hill writes, "Desire is the starting point of all achievement, the first step to all riches." We owe it to our kids to do all we can to open their minds to their own possibilities.

If financial questions are what's holding you back from taking your child to an orthodontist, then you should be aware that there are many creative ways to finance your child's orthodontics, and I'll talk more extensively about that topic in a later chapter. But please don't let concerns about paying for braces stop you from getting them, whether they're for you or for your child. Don't settle for a second-class life because you don't have a first-class smile.

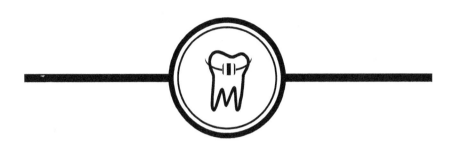

CHAPTER 3

"WHEN SHOULD MY CHILD SEE AN ORTHODONTIST?"

A s I discussed previously, early detection of orthodontic problems is key to getting them fixed quickly and easily, and can prevent small issues from becoming large issues down the line. The American Association of Orthodontists suggests that it's best to get the child in by age seven for an evaluation, because at that stage of growth the child's biology is on our side, and makes intervention easier and faster.

I've seen situations in which parents put off making that initial visit and their children, who'd clearly had issues with crowding, didn't get in to see us until they were twelve or thirteen. In those instances, instead of us trying to expand the arches to create spaces, we had to resort to extraction. We had to remove four permanent teeth from one particular child, because the time had passed and we couldn't regain any of the space that he lost from baby teeth falling out, as all the permanent teeth had already come in.

When we do get the children in early and we can follow the exfoliation of primary teeth, sometimes we can save the excess space that is available in the back because the primary molars are often larger than the permanent premolars that are going to replace those teeth. That means we can hold that space, or use that extra space, to compensate for the child's mouth being crowded. Unfortunately, if we lose that time, we end up losing that space, and we can't regain it—which is when we're forced to perform extractions.

Some scenarios really demand early intervention to correct without significant difficulties. The most difficult malocclusion to treat is a class III malocclusion; with these in particular, you want to start as early as possible, getting the child into some type of reverse headgear or a face mask to try to encourage growth or forward movement of the maxilla so we can correct the malocclusion early. If you don't correct these early enough, ultimately the child will have to undergo jaw surgery. While not every case of this kind can be corrected early, you want to keep the ones that you can from progressing to the point that they'll require either extractions or surgery later in life.

Another scenario in which early intervention is important is when a child is suffering from a breathing problem (which may be exacerbated by severe allergies), to which the parents aren't paying close attention. The child will tend to breathe through the mouth, which has an effect on his or her growth projections. Now that he's constantly hanging his mouth open, the jaw is moving back, so it starts growing more in a vertical direction, which can also cause severe malocclusion. This can result in extensive orthodontic treatment and/or surgery later on in life. Often an orthodontist can catch this early and start the child with an expansion appliance or something along those lines to open the airways if the child has a constricted airway, and/or refer the child to an ENT if it's allergy related. Changing the child's breathing pattern will change their projection and direction of growth.

We discussed crossbite a little in Chapter 1, where the upper teeth fit on the inside of the lower teeth. This is often connected to breathing habits where the upper arch is very constricted or narrow, so the occlusion is totally off. This is another condition that can lead to the need for corrective surgery down the line if it's not corrected early.

Oftentimes aesthetic reasons are what prompts a parent to bring a child in. Either they have severe crowding that's evident early, or they have lots of spacing and/or flaring of the front teeth, and those are obvious things that must be corrected. These may not require orthodontic appliances at the time, but instead what we call "serial extractions," in which the dentist takes out some primary teeth to allow the permanent teeth to correct themselves.

In one situation, I was seeing a ten-year-old boy who had a younger sister with fairly severe flaring of her upper front teeth. He had gotten started in early treatment, but his sister was only five or six-years-old and the parents felt they weren't ready to bring her in at that time. The very next week I saw the family and learned that the little girl had broken her two front teeth. She was simply walking along, not paying attention, when she turned her head and walked into a wall, snapping her two front teeth in half. Had that flaring been corrected, this would never have happened. Her front teeth were vulnerable, having no support.

A CHILD'S GROWING MOUTH

When children are still growing, their jaws and teeth are still developing, so you're able to slowly expand the arch, and the bone basically fills in on the opposite side from where pressure is applied. When this expansion is going on, everything is molding and moving as it normally would, so putting this slight pressure on the bone causes it to remodel. We can encourage the jaws and teeth to grow in the direction we want them to, and use biology to our advantage. If you have a child who has a constricted airway, just expanding that upper arch (maxilla) causes a widening of the airway, because the floor of the nose is at the palate. As we expand the palate, the floor of the nose is also expanding, which increases the size of the airway, allowing the trajectory of growth to change.

As we get older and stop growing, the bone gets denser as it fills in, so it requires more pressure to move teeth. When children come in to see us much later than they should have, we're often going to have to resort to extractions or surgery to get the desired results.

AND DON'T FORGET THE SOCIAL ASPECTS . . .

It's ugly, but it's a fact of life: a child with visibly misaligned teeth grows up being picked on and teased—and the emotional scars and low self-esteem this creates are often bigger problems than the physical issues. If you don't correct misaligned teeth early, children will go through life thinking that they're "less than," that they're "not as good as," or that they can't pursue certain things because they don't feel great about themselves and they're not confident in who they are.

We work with a nonprofit called *Smiles Change Lives*, a program for economically disadvantaged families who can't afford orthodontics. We do the orthodontic work for free for these children, and they're required to write us a letter in the application to explain why they think they should be chosen for this program. In the past few months I've read several letters. One in particular that stood out was from a young lady who admitted that she didn't feel good about herself, and never wanted to smile. Her letter said, "Please choose me to be one of your *Smiles Change Lives* patients, because I feel like if I get my teeth fixed, it would make my life better. I won't be ashamed to try out for stuff, or be ashamed to pursue my goals, or to even set goals, because right now I feel ashamed. I feel like any time I talk people are looking at my mouth, and I try to hide my teeth at all time." These kinds of issues don't go away in adulthood, they just become a part of your worldview, and how you see yourself.

In addition to that, treatment for adults takes longer and is more expensive than treatment for children. It's not just because of the orthodontics that treatment is expensive, it's also because all of the additional work that will have to be done in conjunction with the orthodontics. For instance, if, as a child, an adult patient had a malocclusion, or if they had crossbite, by now they've worn their teeth down unevenly, or they've chipped several teeth because of their teeth misalignment, so, subsequently, they require crowns and veneers in addition to braces. If because of the malocclusion they have developed gum issues, they are likely to need gingival surgery. All of this can wreak havoc on the dentition, the longer the malocclusion stays in place.

THE TWO PHASES OF ORTHODONTICS

When we see children who are between the ages of seven and nine, their orthodontics treatment will usually only last for about twelve to eighteen months at the longest. In these cases, we're looking for problems like crossbites, or permanent teeth that aren't coming in the way they should or when they should. When we see lots of crowding in the primary teeth, or in the mixed dentition, or when we see very narrow arches contributing to crowding and crossbites, those are things we want to address and correct early on. Those patients are put into in what we call a phase one treatment.

In a phase one treatment, we move to correct the problems that exist at that point, then subsequently put the child in some type of retention device until the rest of the permanent teeth have come in. During the time between phase one and phase two, we monitor the child's progress and we see the patient about every three to six months to make sure the permanent teeth are coming in and no other problems are cropping up.

Sometimes the child needs to move onto phase two, but there are many times that continuing treatment beyond phase one is not necessary. If all the permanent teeth come in as they should with adequate spacing, and there's no rotation and no crowding, then we just say goodbye and only see them for retainer visits approximately once a year until growth has ceased. At least 50 percent of our young patients do need to go on to phase two after phase one is completed. When it's the appropriate time, and when we have enough permanent teeth in, then we will commence phase two treatment, after which they will be placed in the retention phase.

WHAT PARENTS SHOULD LOOK FOR

- When upper teeth are sitting behind lower teeth, whether it's in the front, sides, or back. This is known as a crossbite.

- Habits such as thumb and tongue sucking. If you've observed that your child habitually sucks his or her thumb or tongue, then they definitely need to see the orthodontist so this habit can be nipped in the bud before it causes real, lasting damage.

- Permanent teeth that are growing in the wrong spot, such as behind baby teeth that don't seem to be falling out.

- Protruded front teeth, which puts the patient at increased risk for injury or damage, and can cause your child to be teased about their appearance.

- Severe crowding in primary and/or permanent teeth.

- Permanent teeth that are coming in at odd angles through the gums.

- If you have a child with emotional concerns, or a child who simply says, "I don't like my smile."

This last one is a lot more important than you might think, because often you don't know what your child is going through. You may have a child who may only mention it once, then never say another word about it because they think you're not concerned about it, even though it's really bothering them.

We had a mother and her daughter, Janice, who came in for a consultation only because the dentist suggested that they do so.

When we were performing the exam, I asked Janice, "What don't you like about your teeth?"

To her mother's astonishment, Janice replied, "Well, I don't like this, and I don't like that, because the kids call me names at school." Her mother's jaw dropped; she'd never heard about that. It's amazing how often this happens, because I think children can almost be protective of parents, not wanting to worry them.

I know this because it's happened in my own family. My child always wants to make it seem like everything is okay, even when it's not. Sometimes that message could be coming from a parent: "Oh, that's no big deal. Toughen up. Don't worry about what the kids say." But that's easier said than done.

There was an adult woman that I treated who was literally in tears when we took her braces off. She was crying because she just couldn't believe how great her teeth looked and how wonderful she felt after having spent her whole life with an awful-looking bite. When we were taking pictures of her after the removal of her braces, she said, "I never thought I would ever get my teeth fixed. You all don't know how much this means to me. I'm just so overwhelmed." Honestly, I nearly cried, too!

IF YOUR DENTIST TELLS YOU THAT YOUR CHILD NEEDS TO SEE THE ORTHODONTIST . . .

. . . that means now, not a year from now. Even if they've already seen the orthodontist for that initial assessment in the past, and you were told at that time that no treatment was necessary, this doesn't mean after a year or two passes we won't eventually need to intervene. In other words, if you see the orthodontist when your child is seven and you're told then there is no need for intervention, you should still go in for an evaluation about every six to twelve months, just to make sure that everything is continuing to develop as it should.

Remember—when it comes to taking your child to the orthodontist—sooner is better, cheaper, faster, and easier.

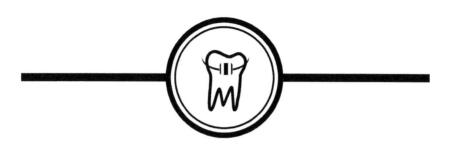

CHAPTER 4

"CAN ADULTS GET BRACES?"

"Oh, my gosh!" That was all I could say when I got my first look at the inside of Ariel's mouth.

"Pretty bad, huh?"

"Well, I had no idea," I had to answer. And that was a little embarrassing, considering she'd worked at the front desk of my office for several months.

You know how people say, "Sometimes you can't see what's right under your nose?" I like to think of myself as a fairly observant person, but when Ariel came to me to say she'd like me to examine her teeth, I was surprised. Why was she considering orthodontics? Looking back, I realized that although she had a very pretty smile, she never showed her teeth. I'd just assumed she was a little shy. Of course, I performed an assessment for her, and when I got her in the chair I was blown away. I never knew that she had the degree of orthodontic problems that she did! Remember, I had never seen her teeth.

When we put Ariel's braces on, she was in tears. She confided that she'd wanted to have her smile corrected all her life, but she had never been able to do so. Now that she had braces on, it was like a lifelong dream was coming true. She thanked me profusely and gave me a big hug—and I'm thinking, you haven't even seen the results yet! In her mind, that was just fine, because she knew she was on her way to getting the smile of her dreams.

What made it even more interesting was that she was a twin, and her sister suffered with the same bite issues. She also came in for a smile assessment, but decided to put off getting her braces. Meanwhile, Ariel was seeing rapid improvements in her smile. Several months into her treatment, Ariel's teeth were looking so much better. I asked her, "Is your sister becoming envious of your smile?"

She said, "Oh, yes, she is! She's going to come in to get *her* braces put on." And she did shortly thereafter. Now they both have gorgeous smiles.

Often the adults who bring their children to us bring them because they themselves suffered criticism or cruel teasing as children because of their smiles. They tell me, "I don't want my child to go through what I had to go through." Once they've seen the changes in their child's smile, I often get these parents as patients, too, when they decide to come in for treatment for themselves. At the time of this writing, within the past couple of weeks, I've seen two or three parents who said, "You might not remember me—you did my child's work several years ago and now I'm ready to get my teeth done."

Sometimes they wait to get started in treatment until their child's work is completed, other times I've put parent and child in braces at the same time.

Yes, adults can get braces, and yes, the positive impact they report on their careers and personal lives is tremendous. I can honestly say I have never had a patient who has regretted getting treatment. Suddenly, they're not shy about doing presentations or smiling at coworkers. It can change everything, because it provides them with a boost in their confidence like nothing else. One patient of mine had always avoided doing presentations at work, and felt as though this really held her career back, so she finally decided to come in for orthodontic treatment. Once her teeth were straight, her self-esteem zoomed, and she told me she was very thankful because she felt like she could be a lot more confident about speaking to people, and was getting more sales.

Another woman brought her daughter to see me. The mom wanted to have straight teeth since she was a child herself, but now she felt she was too old. I told her there was no such thing as "too old for braces," and urged her to at least consider it. She had a lot of spacing issues, and she had an open bite where her teeth didn't overlap. She finally decided to go for it, and we closed the spaces, fixed her bite, and her teeth were just gorgeous. When I saw her last year, she said, "You probably don't remember, but you talked me into getting braces. That was the best decision I could've made. I'm so much happier now about my smile and my bite." Since then, she has sent her sister in to my practice, and her sister's child. When I met her sister, she commented, "We love her new smile. Now it's *my* turn."

DO YOU EVER STOP CARING ABOUT HOW YOU LOOK?

Every so often an adult will tell me they've always wanted braces, but now they feel that they're "too old." That always makes me wonder: is there really a point at which you stop caring about how you look?

I would say no. As long as you're still brushing your hair and washing your face in the morning, you do still care, and an investment in your looks is worthwhile. Believe it or not, a lot of people still think that braces are only for children, and even though they may have wished for years that they could do something to correct the orthodontic problems they have, they think maybe they're too old. Things are better now than they were when I was starting out in my career; I've been in practice for twenty years now, and back when I began, I often had to talk patients into braces, because even if they came in for the consultation they still felt "too old" and worried that others would think they were vain or silly. Maybe getting braces would make them seem as though they were trying to look younger.

Fortunately, a lot of those ideas are no longer generally held, as braces for adults have become more commonplace. These days, if I even have to have that conversation, I point out to them, "Well, apparently, you've thought about it. That's why you're here today. So, there's no need to continue to think about it. The next best time to act is now." Yes, maybe they could have or should have done it years ago—but that's no reason to continue to put it off. *Now* is the best time to make the decision to correct the problem you know you want corrected. We have patients in their sixties; in fact, I put my own mother in braces when she was sixty. Today she's seventy-seven and still wearing her retainers at night.

In 2012, the American Association of Orthodontists reported that 1.2 million adults in the US and Canada received orthodontic treatment, compared to 4.5 million children under seventeen during that same time period. Even celebrities are doing it, too. Singer Faith Hill wore braces at the Grammys in 2013, and she was forty-five at the time. Tom Cruise wore braces at age forty.

Today, about 40 percent of my patients are adults, people who always wanted to change their smile but couldn't afford it earlier in life, or who weren't aware of the changes in technology that have simplified and streamlined treatment. They come in for a lot of different reasons, sometimes because their dentist sends them. This was the case with one patient I had who was getting bridge work done but needed some teeth moved into a better position, because when you put restorative work on teeth that are not properly aligned, there's a greater chance of failure of the restoration. It's better to move teeth to the most optimal position possible to ensure a successful restoration. A lot of times, people will look in the mirror and say, "You know what? I've had crooked teeth all my life," or they have put their children through braces and now decide, "It's my turn. I've always wanted this done, and I'm going to get it done now." Sometimes it's their husband or wife who suggests it.

Life-changing circumstances sometimes push people to make that choice. Career changes, divorce, death of a spouse—these are all reasons that bring patients into our offices saying, "I need to reinvent myself." They get new hairstyles, or change their hair color. They start working out at the gym so they can become more fit. Correcting their smile is just one of those changes they're ready to make.

I have a male patient who is now in his fifties. When we first met, his teeth were so crowded that I wasn't sure how he managed to go as long as he had without getting work done. His bite was awful.

As I write this, he's been in treatment about eight months and we have eliminated most of the crowding. His face and his smile look totally different, and we're not even close to being finished. I think it was during the second visit after we put his braces on that he told me, "It's amazing—my teeth are already changing!"

People will invest in all kinds of things to make themselves look younger and more attractive—but even a facelift isn't going to last as long as a great smile. Simply wearing a retainer will accomplish the preservation of a great smile.

IT'S NOT JUST ABOUT AESTHETICS.

There are solid health reasons to get your bite corrected, in addition to the obvious aesthetic reasons. It's so much easier to keep teeth and gums healthy and clean when they're not so crowded. Good alignment even helps prevent joint and stomach problems, believe it or not. If you can't chew your food correctly, then you end up with stomach issues because you can't digest the food that you're swallowing.

It's true that there are some advantages in terms of the biology of tooth movement when we're working with younger patients, but the difference is so nominal that nobody considering treatment as an adult should worry about it. While children are generally more adaptable, and their lesser bone density means we can move teeth more quickly, adults respond very well to treatment as well. Sometimes I'm asked if there is an age at which it's no longer possible to have braces. My answer is always a resounding, "No, there is not." I have a patient who's about seventy-six now, but he's young at heart. He's very active in his fraternity, and his wife is equally active in her sorority. They travel a lot and golf a lot, and are very sociable. He just wants to look and feel good about himself.

It helps, too, that braces are a lot better looking than they used to be—and some are virtually invisible. A number of adults, especially adults who wore braces when they were children, aren't so anxious to go back in braces, and want to know, "What other options do I have?" Many times they've heard about Invisalign, and want to explore that possibility. I talk more extensively about this product throughout this book, but Invisalign is not actual braces; they are removable, see-through aligners. With aligners, we can correct spacing and crowding without the patient having to wear braces. The best part is they really are nearly invisible, and of course, it's a lot more comfortable. It's also very convenient, because the aligners can be easily removed for whatever reason by the patient, then popped right back in again.

However, not every patient is a good candidate for aligners, because sometimes they have a problem that's a little more involved, so they'll need actual braces or a combination of the two. For those who have aesthetic concerns, we can put them in clear braces, with colored brackets that blend better with the color of their teeth. You don't really see the actual braces unless you're close to the person. The only thing you can see is the wire that connects them. There are even some aesthetic or coated wires available, so that if the patient had to go on stage and give a big presentation and they didn't want the metal wires showing, we could put coated wires on those braces so they are virtually invisible.

Lingual braces—braces that go on the tongue side of the teeth— are also a possibility for people who are concerned about the appearance of braces, and who are good candidates for them. Sometimes problems can be corrected with just a retainer, depending on how minimal the problem is.

PATIENTS WHO COULDN'T HAVE BEEN HELPED IN THE PAST CAN BE HELPED NOW.

Even challenging cases can be successfully treated in adults. One woman's case stands out for me, because it was so clear that getting braces was a life-altering experience for her. When Heather came to us, her teeth and bite were really bad. She'd been a thumb-sucker as a child, and you couldn't even tell she had top teeth if she opened her mouth or if she was talking to you. I knew that more than one doctor said to her, "This can't be corrected without surgery," but we were up for the challenge because she was not interested in surgery, nor could she afford it.

When we took Heather's braces off, she cried. I don't mean she teared up a little—she sobbed like a child. She said that fixing her teeth had totally changed her life. She'd never thought she would be happy about her smile. She even cried as we took her "after" photos—but they were tears of absolute joy. Working on cases such as Heather's makes my work so deeply satisfying; it's terrific to see how fixing someone's smile can totally change how they feel about themselves.

Sometimes adults have issues with missing teeth that have made it more difficult to correct their bites. But now there are mini screws, mini anchors, and other aids that allow us to treat these patients. Before mini anchors became popular, if an adult had missing molars, it was almost impossible to get any anchors in the back of the mouth to which we could attach braces. Now we can just place a mini implant there, and we have our anchor. So many things are possible now that didn't used to be—and chances are they cost a lot less than you think.

For a typical adult who needs bite correction—someone with lots of crowding or excessive spacing—he or she is probably looking at anywhere from two-and-a-half to three years in braces to get their teeth where they need to be. The biggest challenge for my adult patients comes when braces are first put on, because adults seem to have a more difficult time adapting to braces than children do. In fact, I remember one adult woman who was so uncomfortable she asked me to remove her braces. Fortunately, I talked her out of it, and within a week or so she was laughing about that conversation, and thanked me for talking her out of it. Her smile has changed a lot, and she's thrilled about her decision to continue her treatment.

For an adult, adapting to braces typically takes about two weeks. And it's usually after the first visit that my adult patients tell me, "You know what? I don't even think about them anymore." There is some initial discomfort when braces are first put on, but nothing that can't be dealt with by using over-the-counter pain medication, which alleviates the soreness. I think the fact that a lot of adults have difficulty getting used to braces has much to do with an adjustment in the kinds of foods they eat and how they eat them. But, again, people adjust fairly quickly, and soon those new habits become second nature.

My front desk associate, Ariel, has learned how to smile now, and it's lovely to see. She talks a lot more than she used to, and you can see her new confidence in how animated she is in conversations when she used to be more timid. She's my best advertisement!

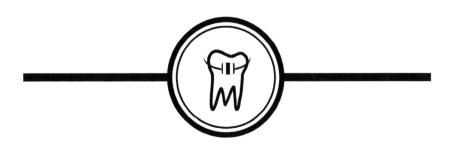

CHAPTER 5

WHAT TO EXPECT ON YOUR FIRST VISIT

"Good morning! Welcome to White Brown Smiles. Let's get your paperwork started—but first, can I get you some coffee?"

We believe first impressions matter, and your first visit to our offices should make you feel like a welcome guest. While not every orthodontic practice is as ardent about greeting both new and regular patients as we are, you should expect to be treated with friendliness, helpfulness, and courtesy, no matter where you go. A good front desk staff tells you a lot about a practice (and so does a front desk staff that's not so great!). We're quite proud of ours.

When you come for your first visit to our offices, you'll be handed paperwork to notify our practice about your past medical history, what brought you to our office, your contact information, and other basic information. Our offices offer the opportunity to fill out much of this information online, saving you some time when you come in. If you're there as the parent of a child seeking treatment, your child will be getting his or her initial x-rays done while you fill out the paperwork; one x-ray will be a panoramic x-ray and the other is a craniofacial x-ray known as a cephalogram, so the doctor can view these x-rays prior to performing your child's smile assessment.

Next, our treatment coordinator will give you a tour of our facilities and answer any preliminary questions you might have. We're used to the sights and noises we hear every day at the office, but we recognize it can be a bit overwhelming for a newcomer, particularly if they're nervous. So, the tour is a welcome icebreaker for most people, and a good way to get a ground-level view of what happens in our offices. It calms a lot of the free-floating anxiety most patients feel on that initial visit, and that's important to us. We love questions, too—and children and adults alike are encouraged to ask as many as they want to.

The treatment coordinator gets to know you; if you or your child has any concerns about treatment, where you heard about our practice, and whether you were referred to us or self-referred. At the end of the tour, they hand you a welcome gift and a card from our practice. Then you'll be escorted to the room where you'll be meeting the doctor and having your initial evaluation.

Our treatment coordinator lets me know you're ready for your assessment, and also lets me know anything they might have learned in talking with you about special concerns or questions. She'll bring me to you, and introduce us. Then she'll go over your stated concerns again with us both, so that if you have anything to add or explain everyone can be brought up to speed.

At that point, I'll perform the patient's assessment, and after, the exam is done and notes are taken, I'll talk to the patient (and parent) about what some of the findings are. I'll pull up the x-rays at the same time and if there are findings on the x-rays I'll point those out. Then, I'll talk you through what I see as the ideal plan of treatment for your or your child's case, referring back to your objectives as I explain.

Sometimes, there's more than one potential treatment plan that could work for a particular patient. If that's the case, I'll walk you through those options, help you make a decision on which treatment modality to go with and also what type of appliances you are going to be using during the treatment. We don't expect our patients to show up primed with all the latest information about what's available—that's our job—and I'll take as much time as necessary to explain all of the possibilities so you can make an informed decision based on what's going to be the best long-term choice for you.

When you've had all of your questions thoroughly answered, the treatment coordinator will take you into their office where they'll break down the cost of treatment and your options for payment. If you decide to go ahead with treatment at that point, and if your dental health is otherwise good and you don't need to see a dentist before you begin, then you'll have the option of getting your treatment started right then and there. This is a boon for our busy patients and parents, because it saves them having to make yet another appointment to begin treatment.

How easy do we make that initial visit for you? One story that sticks in my mind involves a woman named Mary, who came in for an orthodontic assessment for her son, Charles. They went through the entire consultation with the treatment coordinator and me, and at the end of our examination, Mary said she had never experienced such a warm, friendly, and stress-free, first appointment at any medical or dental office in her life. She said she felt welcomed and comfortable—not only in the exam, but with everyone she came into contact with. She expressed how this was a pleasant experience, and one she would never forget. Needless to say, Charles started treatment that very day. Mary's comments are by no means unusual; we get rave reviews from our patients on a regular basis.

And that's how it should be. Patients at our practice, or in any orthodontic practice, should expect to be treated warmly; the atmosphere should be inviting and comfortable, and at the same time highly professional. Your doctor should be willing to answer any questions you have, and be more than willing to explain any diagnosis and recommendation she makes. We want our patients to understand that we value and respect them, which is one of the reasons why we take some time to get to know the patient prior to jumping in and saying, "Okay, let's do an exam."

We make the effort to get to know the patient a little better— to connect on a human level about things such as hobbies, sports, or whatever your or your child's interests are. Again, this is a good way to get younger or nervous patients to relax and begin to feel at home. In all of this, we're setting the stage for our continuing relationship, doing as much as we can to make sure you're comfortable with everything and everyone you'll be seeing, because it's such a long-term relationship; it's not a place where you're going to come in and have one procedure done and you may not go back, it's an ongoing, multi-year commitment, so you want to be very comfortable with the people who you're going to be in a relationship with.

As a patient, you have a right to expect that your concerns and questions will be listened to and answered, and that you'll be treated with respect every step of the way. If you're not clear about why I'm recommending a particular treatment, then you have a right to have that choice explained until it's clear to you.

I've had patients come to me after a less-than-optimal experience in other practices who've reported feeling rushed or brushed off by staff who didn't seem to care whether they were there or not. That's not how we do things, and in my opinion, that isn't the way any patient should be treated at any practice. If you feel as though the doctor isn't really listening to you when you're explaining what your goals are for treatment, that's not a good sign.

Sometimes patients who've done some research come in having already made up their minds about what kind of appliances they want. I get it—maybe a friend of yours reported great results with a particular mode of treatment and you want the same thing, or perhaps you read up about it on the Internet. My job is to really listen to what the patient wants to accomplish and address those things. This is where the dialogue comes in, where the communication comes in, and where the trust comes in when I take the time to explain, "That's not the best choice for you in this case, because . . ." While I'll always do my best to give you what you want, it's more important that you get what you need—because the result is what ultimately matters, not the route we took to get to it, and your friend's situation may be very different from yours.

This is where having established our early rapport is important. I usually find that if these things are explained, utilizing visual props to show the patient why they may need to go in a slightly different direction to gain the ultimate outcome they want, people understand and are more willing to accept my recommendations. That's why we designate about an hour and a half to the new patient consultation, because you just don't know how many questions the patient will have. It's a good idea, by the way, to write down any questions that occur to you before your consultation and to bring that list in with you, since it's easy to forget your questions in the moment. Of course, after patients leave the office, they'll eventually have questions that will come up, but by the time you leave, you will have a contact name and number for the treatment coordinator. You can always call the treatment coordinator back. We have a lot of the most commonly asked questions and answers posted on our website. And of course, the American Association for Orthodontists has a website, too: Braces.org. They have a wide variety of articles and patient information you can read through. Once you've decided to start treatment, we'll either do a scan or take an impression of your teeth.

YOUR VISIT SHOULD BE PLEASANT, NOT ANXIETY PROVOKING.

Patients often come in expecting this process to be an ordeal, and are pleasantly surprised and relieved by how easy, comfortable, and informative the experience is. It's hard not to feel at home when the staff is as bubbly and cheerful as ours is. There are plenty of adults out there who don't much relish the idea of having their teeth worked on, and some people are downright terrified. But I find that sitting down with them and talking through their thoughts and fears can be quite calming, and helps them feel more so as if they're in the driver's seat of the process.

This isn't a dentist's office where there's drilling and filling going on; our processes are far less stressful. In the orthodontic office, a typical appointment is changing a wire, or simply adjusting your braces. You're not coming in for a shot. You're not going to be numbed. A lot of times, once patients hear that, their fears evaporate and they relax.

Believe it or not, a lot of people come in thinking that getting braces is invasive and painful (it's not!). They assume they will get numbing shots or even need to be put to sleep, because they think it's going to be painful. But once we let them know how the braces are applied and show them models with braces on, they're on board and eager to start the process. And, like most orthodontics practices, we charge no fee for that initial exam and consultation. That alone is a great reason to make an appointment, so you can get questions answered and look into getting that smile you've always wanted.

Sometimes patients will ask me, "Are there any guarantees?" Well, I can't guarantee that you're going to have a smile like Julia Roberts. But something unique we offer is a lifetime guarantee. If your teeth shift because you weren't wearing your retainers and you have to get back in braces for a short period of time, we'll put you back in braces. When you're done with treatment and fitted with a retainer, we do stress the importance of consistently wearing your retainer to keep your teeth where you want them. But sometimes, even patients with the best of intentions don't wear their retainers, or maybe they lose or break them, and just don't get around to having them replaced. Then, over time, your teeth will naturally begin to shift back to where they were before you wore braces. We don't want that to happen. Fortunately, patients who see shifting are quick to come back and have it corrected—and the sooner they do, the less time they'll have to spend in braces again. It doesn't take a full mouth of braces to get things back in position, it just takes brackets on the teeth that have shifted for about three months to realign those teeth. Then we put them back in retainers and send them on their way. Very, very occasionally, something can change once we're in treatment. We are, after all, dealing with the body, not a machine, and sometimes things will crop up unexpectedly. For instance, something could go wrong with a tooth; you might lose an old filling, get sent to the dentist, and be told that it can't be saved. Then you'd need an extraction, and that could change your treatment plan somewhat, depending on how the body adapts to that change. This is rare however, and if you've been to the dentist before starting treatment (as you should), there should be few surprises.

Usually what I find in meeting patients is that the person has already pretty much made up his or her mind to go ahead with the process and get their smile corrected. No one just shows up arbitrarily at the orthodontist's office; when they come in for the appointment, they are there because they want to be helped with a problem they perceived they have, whether they'd been told about said problem, or whether they discovered it on their own. But they come in wanting our help, and our job is to give them all the information and help them make the decision they know they want to make.

One little girl, about age nine, came in very nervous about getting braces. We did her smile assessment and went over everything with her mom and her, with the girl asking us questions a mile a minute. When it was time for her to get her braces, she got in the chair still firing off questions—and we were still answering them. I could see that just talking through all of this was making her fears subside—and they certainly did, because she was so relaxed at that point, she fell asleep in the chair! She was sleeping so hard that when I was finished I literally had to shake her, because just calling her name did not wake her up. I often share that story with my clinicians, because it's a real testimony to you when your patient falls asleep in your chair. They have to be very relaxed to do so.

If you're taking your child to an orthodontist, it's important that your doctor is comfortable and experienced working with children. Orthodontists are people, too; some of them can create a good rapport with both young people and adults, while others tend to be best with young people, and some would prefer to work mostly with adults. A patient is looking for a well-rounded person with a good personality and a good attitude—a "people person." If they're a people person, then they can get on a child's level and talk about sports, or about piano lessons, or about whatever the child is into. It's fine if they don't know much about the topic, because children love to feel like they're teaching an adult. That's how to build rapport with them. They feel very special. Building a relationship with a child is just as easy as building one with an adult; it just takes getting to know them and dealing with them as people. Then they feel like they're part of the family. With two lively young sons of my own, I'm very comfortable working with children.

Everything about your initial visit should make you feel comfortable, safe, and welcome. You should leave understanding exactly what will be done, what the timetable is, what it will cost, and how you'll be paying.

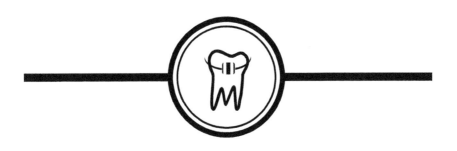

CHAPTER 6

NEW OPTIONS AND TREATMENTS

"Oh, my gosh—my daughter had it so much harder! Josh doesn't know how easy he has it!" Alicia saw both of her children go through orthodontic treatment, and her amazement at the changes made in the science of tooth movement in just those few years says everything about the rapid strides we're making in technology in the field of orthodontics.

With her daughter, Sophia, the first of the two children we treated, we used traditional metal braces with the tie wings. She also had to have an expander, a device that creates room in the upper arch and widens it. These were the standard treatments at the time, and they really weren't comfortable. But by the time her brother,

Josh, was ready for his braces, we'd just started using the Damon self-ligating braces, which have little sliding gates on them that do not require a tie. We used special copper NiTi wires with these braces, which are constantly moving the teeth, whereas the previous generation of wires moved to a certain point and then stopped. We did not have to use an expander, which is the widening appliance, on Josh. Sophia was in retainers at that point. They both ended up with a beautiful smile, but Josh had a much easier and more comfortable orthodontic experience.

Thankfully, braces aren't what they used to be. New advances in the science of orthodontics have made the process much less uncomfortable and intrusive.

These are the basic kinds of braces/brackets we use today:

- **Traditional metal brackets:** Stainless steel or titanium with tie wings. We use elastic ties to secure the wire in the bracket.

- **Self-ligating braces:** These brackets have little doors. You don't have to tie the wire in, so the wire is free to move in the slot. Therefore, less pressure has to be applied to move teeth. In this system, you have less resistance which provides more efficient movement of the teeth.

- **Aesthetic brackets:** Clear or tooth-colored brackets. These come in either the traditional style or in a self-ligating style, and help to make braces less noticeable.

- **Incognito braces:** Braces placed behind the teeth, or lingual braces. This is another aesthetic treatment modality. They're nearly invisible because they're behind the teeth on the tongue side so no one sees them. These braces are typically one hundred percent customized. We make the molds of the scan, send them to the lab, and the lab manufactures the braces and the wires to fit the individual patient perfectly. Then we just place the braces and wires, as with regular braces. This is a good alternative in cases where the patient can't use Invisalign, but doesn't want to go with clear braces either. They do require additional chair time and special tools, so patients using Incognito generally can expect longer appointments, but treatment time overall should be about the same as with standard braces.

- **Invisalign:** A popular solution that uses clear plastic aligners that are designed to move the teeth incrementally, without brackets or braces. With this system, rather than patients coming in and having brackets applied to their teeth, we make molds or scans of their teeth and send them off to the lab. They create a series of aligners that incrementally move the teeth. You will wear one aligner for two weeks and then progress to the next aligner, wearing that for two weeks. Incrementally, every two weeks, you're creating a different set of movements until you get to that final position. An aligner looks like a clear retainer, and it just snaps on to the teeth. Most adults love Invisalign because it's not intrusive. It's very comfortable. They can take their aligners out and eat, brush, and floss like they normally would if they were not undergoing orthodontic treatment, and that's a huge plus. And it's aesthetically pleasing; it looks like there is nothing on your teeth at all. Most people don't even know that you're wearing Invisalign.

Invisalign now has a product called Invisalign Teen. They come with a slightly higher price tag because they supply you with extra aligners if your teen loses them (and they do, believe me). It also has an indicator dot on the individual aligner, which tells the practitioner whether that patient is actually wearing the aligner as instructed. If the patient has worn that aligner the number of hours he or she should have, then the dot slowly disappears. This provides the orthodontist with a kind of check and balance. Children will typically tell the parent, "I'm wearing it all the time," but when they get to the orthodontist and we see this dot, we can point out, "This dot is very blue. You have not been wearing this aligner." It also allows for teeth to continue to erupt, whereas in adults those teeth aren't still erupting, everything is in place, so they don't have to make that allowance in the aligners.

Why aren't these dots on the adult version of Invisalign? Not surprisingly, adults who are paying for their own work are far more likely to wear their aligners or braces as prescribed. Adults will come in and tell me, "When I was a teenager I didn't wear my retainer. I didn't do anything they told me to do. Now that I'm paying for it, if you tell me to wear my rubber bands twenty-four hours a day, I'm following orders, because now it's my money."

WHO CAN'T USE INVISALIGN?

Invisalign would be counterproductive if the patient's malocclusion were too involved. Let's say the patient has a tremendous amount of crowding and needs teeth removed; that case is a little more involved than Invisalign alone can typically correct. Invisalign will only be able to take us so far, and at some point, we will have to attach brackets to the patient's teeth to get them into the optimal position. Discrepancies in the bite are another problem that Invisalign can't correct on its own. For instance, if the patient had a severe crossbite we'd need significant expansion and widening of the arch. Those are cases in which Invisalign is going to be limited in its ability to create the amount of expansion that we may require.

Invisalign users must utilize elastics to help correct open bites. Whether it's from thumb sucking or mouth breathing, if the patient's upper and lower front teeth don't meet or don't overlap Invisalign may close it down to some extent, but at some point, we're going to have to put attachments on these teeth to move them further.

Sometimes I get patients who are eager to use Invisalign, even when it's not the ideal choice for them, so we'll work out a hybrid treatment plan that includes braces as well. We'll give them the pros and cons, and most of the time, when we talk through it, those patients concerned about the aesthetic part of it decide to go with the clear braces. One patient I remember simply couldn't tolerate braces, and after a few weeks she told me, "I just can't do this. I have to do the Invisalign." So, we took her braces off, made molds for Invisalign, and got her Invisalign going. At the end, we had to put brackets in the back to help move some back teeth that Invisalign just couldn't correct adequately. She didn't have a mouth full of braces to finish up, but she did have small sections here and there to get her to the endpoint. She was thrilled with the end result.

I'm not eager to place young children in Invisalign, mostly because they might not wear them as often as they should. In order to be effective, Invisalign must be worn roughly twenty-two hours a day—pretty much any time you're not eating or brushing your teeth, those aligners should be in place. If you have a child who constantly has their aligners out because they're eating and then forget to put them back in, it could end up being a waste of your time and money.

It's going to severely prolong treatment because you won't be getting the movement you should be getting.

The other issue is if you have a child who is too young to be responsible. They constantly lose their aligners, which means it's costing you money twofold. When I'm working with parents, I give them the pros and cons, talk to them about typical scenarios, and then ask them, "Do you think your child is responsible enough?" We do run across the occasional thirteen-year-old who is very responsible, so they may end up in Invisalign if they or their parents insist.

HOW BRACES HAVE CHANGED FOR THE BETTER

Back in the old days, braces used stainless steel wires, and every movement had to be made by placing a bend in the wire. Now, with the advent of brackets that have tip and torque in them, we don't have to bend the wire as often, and the wires themselves are made of different material. Rather than steel, we use nickel titanium wires, which are more flexible, as well as beta titanium and some stainless-steel wires toward the end of treatment.

The next generation of wires is the heat-activated wire. We use this type of wire quite often, because it is constantly moving the teeth, making these wires more efficient than their predecessors. We put the wires in place, and when the wire temperature reaches the patient's body temperature, it's active. The minute the patient drinks a glass of cold water, the wire is deactivated and goes limp, like a cooked spaghetti noodle. When the mouth gets back to normal body temperature, that wire becomes active again. It's constantly activating and deactivating, which is why teeth movement is so much more efficient; you have a constant movement or adjustment of the teeth, whereas if a tooth was slightly out of place and I put a stainless-steel wire on it, there's a tremendous amount of pressure to move that tooth and that pressure is applied all at once. That makes it far more uncomfortable. This new kind of wire is going to move that tooth slowly but more efficiently, as it's in a self-ligating bracket. In other words, it's not tied in, so the wire can freely move around and simply "jiggle" the tooth in place. Thanks to the flexibility of these wires, they're also much less likely to break than their old steel counterparts.

When the patient comes back in for an evaluation, if the wire hasn't leveled out the tooth or the bite as much as we wanted it to, we just take that wire out, allow the wire to go back to its normal shape, and then we retie that same wire. The wire has memory in it—once you take it out, the wire goes back to its normal shape. When you tie it back in, it's distorted again. The wire always wants to come back to its normal position, and that's why you get that consistent movement of the teeth. The doors on the newer brackets make adjustments much easier too—these little "doors" work just like a sliding door, going up or down. When it gets into position, it locks in.

WHEN YOU GO IN FOR YOUR SMILE ASSESSMENT, BRING AN OPEN MIND.

It's probably best not to go in to an initial consultation with an orthodontist with too many preconceived expectations, either in terms of the treatment you want or the results you are trying to achieve. Keep an open mind about what kind of treatment you want, and let the doctor's expertise be the guide. Occasionally, patients will come in with expectations or goals they have set in their mind about how they want their teeth to look that are just not practical. If you are a fifty-year-old adult, you most likely already have worn teeth, uneven edges, and teeth that have recessed. You can't expect to wind up with a smile like a twenty-year-old—there are going to be some differences. Of course, when your orthodontic treatment is complete, you can choose to go to your cosmetic dentist and have some enhancements to get the cosmetic outcome you are after.

That's why good doctor/patient communication is so important—especially in the beginning of the process—so together you can discuss what the possibilities are, what you can do with braces, what you can't do, and what other treatment or procedures might be necessary to get you to where you want to be. Often while I'm doing that initial exam a new patient will ask me, "Can you make my teeth look like yours?"

I have to tell them, "No, I can't make your teeth look like mine. However, we can align your teeth and fix your bite and your teeth will look superb." Your teeth are a certain shape, size, and color, and orthodontics alone can't change that. It's important to talk this over and get patients to a point where they have reasonable expectations.

Cosmetic procedures can be performed to move people a long way closer to the smile they want. We do laser teeth whitening in our office, for instance. We also offer **laser soft tissue treatment** for people whose gums overlap or cover the teeth more than they should. We can do aesthetic gingival contouring to make those properly aligned teeth look even better once we've removed all the excess gum tissue overlapping the teeth. Granted, some people do have shorter clinical crowns than others, but a lot of the time it's just the redundant gum tissue that's hanging over the top third of the tooth that makes the tooth look small. With laser contouring, we can reveal much more of the tooth and really improve the look of your smile. We actually do this process fairly often on children too, especially those who have hygiene issues in which the gums are irritated and growing over their brackets.

We can also use the laser to speed treatment along. Sometimes we see a child with a tooth that's trying to come in but is only partially uncovered. Previously we'd just had to wait it out, or we'd refer the patient to another specialist. These days I just pull out my laser, remove the excess gum tissue, put a bracket on the tooth, and now we can move that tooth in place instead of having to wait six months for it to come down by itself.

Some other recent technology that has made my and my patient's lives easier includes the following:

Temporary Anchorage Devices (TADs) are mini screws that anchor in the bone, and are another relatively recent development in technology that gives us new options in treating both adults and children to help move teeth even more efficiently. Let's say we have an adult who has lost several back teeth, but we need to retract their front teeth. Because the back teeth are gone, we don't have those to use as anchors. But with TADs we just place these mini-anchors and we can move teeth. We use them in children as well because it's a more efficient anchorage device. When you place teeth against teeth, the stronger tooth acts as the anchor and holds things back as the weaker tooth moves toward it. But you still have both teeth moving, so it's kind of like a tug of war. With a mini anchor—once you anchor the mini screw in the bone—the tooth's not moving at all, so it's a lot more efficient when you're trying to move teeth in one direction and you don't want the teeth you're putting it against to move at all.

AcceleDent is another new technology that many orthodontists are employing to speed treatment results. This is a device with a custom mouthpiece. You give this to the patient and they wear it about twenty minutes every day. The device delivers micropulses to speed up tooth movement—almost like massaging the tooth. The movement increases blood flow to the area, which in turn, leads to reparative cells rushing in the area to help with tooth movement.

Another new technology is **Propel**, which helps speed tooth movement with a stubborn tooth. This involves the orthodontist putting a little mini screw in around the roots of the tooth, then removing the screw. By doing this we're creating trauma selectively around the tooth, which triggers a healing process that helps with the tooth movement. With tooth movement, you have bone being destroyed on the pressure side, and new bone being laid down on the tension side. So, when you create this trauma, the influx of reparative cells comes in and aids in that movement.

Imaging scanners are a huge leap forward for patients who hate having those goopy impressions taken—and who doesn't? With the scanner, in just a few minutes we can make a highly detailed, three-dimensional scan of your teeth that can be used as the model for the labs that manufacture whatever devices or appliances your treatment protocol demands.

Thanks to all the great new alternatives available to us, chances are that even if you were told some years ago that your case couldn't be treated, it can be treated successfully now because of advances in technology.

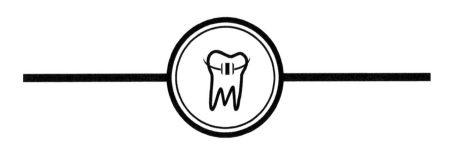

CHAPTER 7

WHAT TO EXPECT IN TREATMENT

Although every case and every patient is different, there *are* some aspects that nearly all of them share—and this chapter is about answering the most common questions I'm asked by people who are just starting out their orthodontic treatment.

HOW IN THE WORLD DO I KEEP THESE BRACES CLEAN?

This is by far the question I hear most often from patients who've just had their braces placed. Of course, it's also the first thing we go through with them after braces are installed: how to keep your or your child's teeth clean, and how to brush and floss properly. Hygiene isn't as tricky as it may look when you first see your braces on, but it will take a little more time and effort than you may be used to since you now have more surface area to brush around. It's going to take a little extra time to floss too, because now you must clean under the wire. Although it's daunting at first, after a few days it will become routine.

Many of my patients decide to invest in "power tools" to help them clean their teeth. When parents ask me for recommendations, I tell them that whatever will get their child more excited about good oral hygiene and will keep them brushing is probably a good investment. Some patients use an oscillating electric toothbrush, which helps them do a more thorough job at brushing around the braces and around the wires. A Waterpik is also very helpful; this is a tool that shoots pulsing jets of water out of its tip to dislodge food particles, sort of an electric flosser. It gets back into hard-to-reach areas that people often miss with regular flossing. Flossing aids (non-electric) help to thread the floss under the wire so that patients can more easily floss their teeth while they're in braces. I find power toothbrushes and Waterpiks are particularly useful for young children who aren't as adept at cleaning their teeth.

Even if your child has been brushing independently, you need to step in at this point and oversee brushing until you're sure your child is doing a thorough job. Your child may not like that initially, but an ounce of prevention is worth a pound of cure—and it's much easier for them to have their teeth inspected by Mom or Dad than to go through the trouble and expense incurred if they don't take proper care of their teeth while they're in braces. Just prepare yourself for some eye rolling.

What happens when you don't clean properly? One of the most common problems is decalcification, which is a demineralization of the enamel itself; this shows up as white spots on the teeth, and is the beginning of the cavity process. When you have food and bacteria sitting on the teeth, the acid the bacteria produce begins demineralizing the enamel, and that's what causes those white spots. We see this frequently in children who don't practice good oral hygiene. It can also lead to periodontal issues when they're not flossing as they should. The tarter build-up that occurs causes the gums to become irritated and puffy, and if the tarter is left there long enough it can start wearing away the bone that supports the teeth.

Often, this kind of scarring can be repaired with restorations—but that's expensive, and it's completely preventable. Why spend all that money on braces if you're going to let your teeth go? You don't want to go through this process to get a beautiful, straight smile, and wind up with scarring on the enamel.

WHAT CAN I EAT WITH BRACES ON?

For the first few days we encourage patients to stick with a soft food based diet, and to stay away from anything that's too hard or too crunchy, because even though the brackets are set, there is a lag time where the final set occurs—approximately twenty-four hours after they're installed—so we do ask them to take it easy up to that point. Softer foods are more manageable than trying to chew a steak the first day you get your braces on, so we advise patients to stick with pasta and potatoes, and soft meats such as chicken and fish.

We definitely tell them to stay away from hard candies and nuts—but usually the challenge with foods is changing the way in which the patient eats them, specifically hard foods like carrot sticks or apples. It's our tendency to bite off pieces of harder foods with our front teeth and then chew with our molars, but biting hard foods in braces—even an apple—can snap a wire or break the bond on the braces. If the patient wants to have an apple, we recommend cutting it into bite-size pieces. Don't just cut the apple in half or in slices and then bite into it, because that creates the same destructive pressure and you'll wind up with broken braces. We ask patients not to bite into sandwiches because the pressures from biting into something can damage the braces. They could bite in to a piece of lettuce or something that's a bit firmer than the meat that's in the sandwich and cause a bracket to become dislodged. Not to mention that once you're in braces, you have to stay away from anything sticky or gummy: Laffy Taffy, sticky candies, caramel apples, or chewing gum that can pull at the braces.

When I put braces on children, I ask them to sign a contract that lays out the rules on what and how they're going to eat. This is intended to emphasize the point that it's their responsibility to stay away from the foods on the "don't eat" list. We also spell out, "Don't put objects in your mouth," because children often have habits like chewing on pencils or pen caps in class. We make sure they understand those are habits they will have to change now that they're in braces. They must also promise to keep their teeth clean when they have braces on because that's going to prevent dental issues such as cavities and decalcification. They sign a pledge to take care of their braces, to keep them clean, and to keep their teeth and gums healthy.

IS IT GOING TO HURT? IF IT DOES, WHAT DO I DO?

In my experience, the pain experienced is mild and not at all comparable to, say, the throbbing pain of a toothache. However, patients in newly installed braces are going to feel some soreness because the teeth are moving and will produce some discomfort when chewing. The initial tenderness or achy feeling should pass within a couple of days, five at the most. Meanwhile, we suggest the patient take what they normally would take if they had a headache: over-the-counter pain medications such as Tylenol (acetaminophen) as needed every four to six hours for pain for at least the first two days. After that, the pain should subside and they typically won't need any medication.

That said, everyone's pain threshold is different, and a lot of times we'll have patients who are worried because, "My friend said that she was in a lot of pain after she got her braces on." Well, that friend may have an unusually low pain threshold, whereas you may have a higher pain threshold and it won't bother you. Everyone's experience is going to be different as far as that's concerned.

HOW OFTEN DO I HAVE TO COME IN FOR OFFICE VISITS?

It used to be that braces had to be checked monthly, but these days you'll be going into the office far less frequently. With the advances in wires and the technology we use today, you only have to be seen every six to ten weeks.

Those office visits will be brief, and usually involve adjusting or changing your wires, or adjusting the elastics. What we do depends on where you are in your course of treatment. When you get a little bit farther along—at the point where you're in stiffer wires—we could be putting bends in the wires, or otherwise adjusting the shape of the wire. The best news is that these appointments are typically quite brief, lasting twenty to thirty minutes at the most, so they're easy to squeeze into a busy schedule.

In the old days of only stainless steel wires, teeth would move to a certain point then you'd have to have your wires changed. But thanks to the advent of the self-ligating systems we discussed in an earlier chapter, these modern, heat-activated wires are more resilient than the old stainless steel wires. Now you have flexible wires that will work over a longer period of time, which is why we don't need to see our patients every month anymore.

WHAT'S THE PERIOD OF ADJUSTMENT LIKE WHEN YOU GET BRACES?

Parents worry that their children will experience a lot of discomfort getting used to braces, or that they won't be able to tolerate having them in their mouth. Interestingly, between adults and children, it's children who adjust more quickly; within a week or two braces seem totally normal to them. Adults can sometimes take longer, and report more initial pain (although nothing that can't be handled with over-the-counter pain medication). But even people who initially find them very challenging get used to them by the second week.

The bigger issues are usually around food, and getting used to the restrictions on what and how you can eat, as outlined previously. Sometimes we do have some challenges with young children who insist on eating anything and everything that they want to. Those children might take a little longer adjusting, not because of the braces, but because of their habits, which may cause their wires to break or come out prematurely. With these children, sometimes there's an adjustment period before they come to the realization that they really need to change their eating habits.

As I've noted, adjustment periods for adults tend to be longer; maybe we're just more stuck in our ways. Occasionally I'll get a patient with an extremely low pain threshold. One lady I worked on actually lost a lot of weight because her teeth were so sore. In response, I put the lightest wires on her and she did much better. We've had some patients we've had to drop down to a smaller wire size to help get them used to the braces before we could move up to the size of wire that we would typically have used with their type of malocclusion.

Sometimes, patients are taking medications that make their mouths dry, so the brackets are rubbing them a little more than they typically would if they didn't have dry mouth. We're likely to see these patients a little more frequently, helping them and talking them through these first few months and getting them used to the braces. We encourage them to keep a water bottle handy and take sips from it throughout the day to keep their mouths moist.

No matter what your age, there's going to be a slight adjustment period; I personally believe a lot of it is just psychological for both adults and children. It's good to realize ahead of time you're going to experience this slight transition so that you can be prepared—but know also that most of the time, within about a month or two, my patients are so used to their braces that they forget they're there. Typically, they tell me, "You know what? I don't even think about them anymore."

Anytime we are made to cope with something that forces us to adjust our habits, we focus on it until the newness wears off. The day you get your braces on (and for a few days after that) it may seem to you that there's no way you're ever going to get used to having this "stuff" in your mouth—but stay focused on your end goal and that beautiful smile you're working toward and it will be much easier. Good goals always require some work on our parts to achieve, and the great news is that—faster than you may think possible the day they're put on—your braces will stop feeling so new and odd, and simply become your new normal.

ARE THERE PROBLEMS I MIGHT EXPERIENCE THAT MEAN I NEED TO CALL MY ORTHODONTIST?

New patients worry about potential problems with their braces, but most of the issues they call us about are just part of the process of getting accustomed to their new braces. If you have pain that over-the-counter medications isn't helping, you might want to call in. Legitimate reasons to call in are things like a wire poking you, or a bracket that's come off. We're always happy to hear from patients and certainly never discourage them from calling us with their questions or concerns, though we do our best to prepare them for what to expect so that none of the normal adjustment issues worry them unnecessarily. We talk them through some home remedies that are helpful: warm saltwater rinses or Peroxyl rinses if things are a little sore, or if the issue is gum irritation. But short of having a broken wire or another technical issue around the braces themselves, you probably wouldn't have to come into the office between appointments.

When I think about patients who go through a particularly tough period of adjustment, one woman comes to mind. Sandra is in her fifties. When she got her braces on, she was acutely uncomfortable that first week. She actually called the office and said, "You know, I think I've made the worst decision of my life. I need to have these braces removed."

The office manager basically talked her down off the ledge and told her, "Just come in if you feel like you need to come in, but give it some time."

She agreed to give it some time—and now whenever Sandra walks into the office she's smiling from ear to ear. She's gone from, "Get these off!" to, "I am so glad she talked me into keeping these on. I don't even realize that they're there anymore. I just love my braces!" She's our biggest fan, and her teeth are already looking much better after just five months of treatment.

Yes, there are some things you'll need to change, new sensations you'll have to become accustomed to, and new habits to make (and old habits to break) when you go into braces. But, like Sandra, you'll get used to the changes much more quickly than you think—and the results will be worth it.

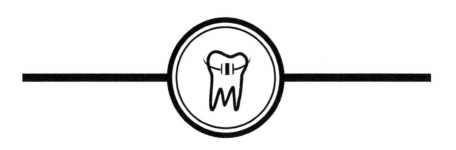

CHAPTER 8

WORKING WITH THE FEARFUL PATIENT

anny was only twelve years old. He looked more like a beefy sixteen-year-old, yet when it came to visiting my office for the first time he was more like a frightened child. Both of his parents came in with him for the initial consultation. Clearly, he needed braces, and after his exam and records were done I put him in the chair.

He didn't stay there long.

The first part of the process of getting braces installed is attaching the brackets to the teeth. It's necessary for the teeth to be thoroughly dry for the adhesive to work, and the tech needs a nice, open mouth to get in there. She put the mouth props on Danny's teeth to hold his jaws open—and he leapt up and snatched them out.

"I can't breathe! You're trying to kill me!"

The clinician looked at him, and looked at me. Now what?

We talked him back into the chair. The clinician showed him a cotton roll.

"We can use this instead, but we have to keep your teeth dry, okay?"

Danny wasn't having it. We tried and tried for an hour, accommodating him in every way we could think of. We let him sit up, we used the minimum number of cotton rolls that we could, and still, every time we put them in he spat them out, insisting that he couldn't stand it and he didn't want braces. Looking back, I think he was probably severely claustrophobic, but at that point I thought it was time to throw in the towel—at least for that session.

I went and got his mom and told her, "I don't think we're going to be able to do this today. It doesn't appear that he's ready for this. We have given it our best efforts, but this is not going to happen today."

His mother looked at me, looked at him, and said in a tone that allowed no contradiction, "Oh yes, we *are* going to do this today." She turned to her son, "Hey, we talked about this. I took the time off. You're out of school. Not one more word. You're going to sit in that chair and let them do what they need to do." We could see by his response that he was used to doing as he was told—and he could see Mom wasn't playing.

Back in the chair for round two. We worked to put just one bracket on at a time, holding his lip away from his teeth with our fingers. Slowly but surely, we were able to at least get one arch on, and put his wire in. Typically installing a whole set of braces takes an hour, but at this point half the day was gone. Everyone was exhausted by lunchtime, including me. I knew Danny was, too.

When he came back for the bottom set, we applied the lower braces in the same slow, painstaking way. We kept him with the same assistant too, because during his previous visit she had managed to earn his trust. Amazingly enough, after about two or three visits, Danny turned into the perfect patient. He actually enjoyed coming to the office, and was all smiles when we saw him. I think he was so afraid of the unknown that he had just psyched himself out.

Claustrophobia is a big contributor to patient discomfort, though patients don't always make that association. One lady who came to see us told us from the beginning that she was claustrophobic and that she couldn't be tilted back in the chair all the way. That meant we had to work on her with her seated at about a forty-five degree angle, because if we tried to put her lower, she couldn't breathe. We took frequent breaks to give her a minute to collect herself, and then we would work again. It's tough for claustrophobic patients—they have intrusive dental props in their mouth, I'm leaning over them, the assistant is leaning over them, and they begin to panic, feeling as though they're going to be smothered. Of course, it's psychological because there is nothing actually obstructing their breathing, but for them, it feels terrifyingly real. For us, the challenge is talking them through it, making the process as comfortable and stress free as it can be while we're getting the work done.

Like Danny, this woman started out as a challenging patient, but once we'd earned her trust she became more comfortable and compliant. In fact, she said when she went to her new dentist, she "laid down the law." She told them, "Going to White Brown Smiles has me spoiled. When I need a break, they give me a break. When I tell them, 'I need to sit up,' they allow me to sit up. So, if you can do that, then you can be my dentist."

One of the procedures in orthodontics that claustrophobic patients have real difficulty with is the taking of dental impressions. We had a young man in recently who snatched the impression tray out of his mouth the moment we put it in. To help alleviate this issue, there are several products that numb the soft palate, so that when a person is claustrophobic or has a hyperactive gag reflex, we can numb those muscles that cause gagging. We also try to use the 3D scanner as much as we can because it eliminates the need for taking impressions, and if we know in advance that a patient can't tolerate the tray we always use it.

WHY ARE CHILDREN SO OFTEN FEARFUL ON THAT FIRST VISIT?

Oddly enough, children report that their fears are most often passed along to them from the adults around them: "Oh, you're going to get a needle." Anecdotally, this kind of remark often comes from someone who's just teasing—but the child is taking it seriously. Not surprisingly, the child freaks out.

The other reason children are often fearful is because of what they've heard from their peers. Sometimes a sibling or schoolmate will tell them, "Oh, it's going to really hurt when you get your braces on." Sometimes the friends know better but they want to scare them. We always make time for the child to ask us any questions they have. If they're shy, sometimes the parent will say, "Don't you want to know whether it's going to hurt or not?" When it's the parent who is posing the question, I can tell there's been some conversation about it. It's at that point we try to ease their fears and assure them that,

"Applying the braces is not going to hurt you." We talk them through different scenarios to let them know exactly what's going to happen and what they can expect, and that's usually enough to get them over their worries.

We had a young child in recently and as we were putting his braces on, I could feel his body trembling. When I see patients like that, I talk to them throughout the entire procedure, letting them know exactly what I'm doing so that there are no surprises: "Okay. I'm going to shine a light. Nothing is going to hurt. All you need to do is just sit there with this mouth prop in, and I'm going to do the rest. You're not going to feel a thing," just constantly speaking in a calming tone to them. After we've done half of the mouth I tell them, "Hey, we're halfway done. You didn't feel anything. Nothing hurt you during that process, and the second half is going to be exactly the same."

Sometimes what kids are scared of isn't actually pain, but that somehow having braces is going to make them the school geek and that they'll be teased. One young lady was highly resistant to the idea of getting braces, and her mother had to tell me that was why. Her mom insisted that she go through with it, and happily at her next visit she was able to report that the other kids didn't tease at all, but were just curious about her new braces. All of the extravagant fears she'd come in with were laid to rest, and she too became a cheerful patient.

Sometimes it's the parent, not the child, who can't handle being in the room while the child's braces are being applied. Usually it's during the initial consultation that I discover who the tense one really is. I remember one mom who was in the consultation with her daughter asking endless questions. I could see that Mom's concerns weren't just surface concerns. She was clearly so anxious that I finally

"EVERYTHING YOU WANT IS ON THE OTHER SIDE OF FEAR."

JACK CANFIELD

came out and asked her, "Mom, you seem to be more nervous than your daughter is. Can we help you with that? What kinds of questions do you have?"

The floodgates opened: "You are so right! I am nervous, because I've never been through this before. I don't want her to be in pain, and I don't want her to be uncomfortable." Once I talked her though the process, she calmed down. Her daughter on the other hand was fine with it from the beginning; she just asked a few questions, and was satisfied when we answered them.

When I'm working with a fearful patient I have a number of ways to help put them at ease. A big part of fear is facing the unknown—so I make sure to speak to them throughout the procedure, describing what I'm doing and what it will feel like so there are no surprises. I make sure they get lots of short breaks, and I keep the atmosphere as light and pleasant as I can. I find that even the most fearful patient can relax when they're treated with sensitivity and thoughtfulness.

WORKING WITH SPECIAL NEEDS CHILDREN

Special needs patients also require extra care and sensitivity to feel comfortable. One of my patients is a young autistic girl. Instead of doing everything in one visit as we would have with the average patient, we put on just four or five brackets at a time, give her a break, and then go back and do another four or five and give her another little break, so she didn't get overwhelmed. It's just a matter of putting enough time on the schedule, being attentive to their needs, and having them let you know when they're ready to proceed.

Special needs patients may also have some difficulty processing and following directions. Sometimes if you ask them to do something they may not completely understand exactly what you're requesting of them. Usually when we're working with these children it's helpful to have the parent sit close by. I find that the parents are usually better than we are at reaching their kids verbally, and often will be able to relay my instructions to the child in language the child can better understand.

TREATING THE ACTIVE CHILD

Some children are in almost constant motion in the chair; they may abruptly sit up in the middle of the procedure, and they wiggle a lot—they just can't stay still and will move their heads around to try to see what you're doing. Again, I find that taking a calming tone is tremendously helpful. One little girl couldn't stop moving her tongue; it seemed to be everywhere at once. We were able to put the mouth prop in, but we couldn't put a bite guard in because her tongue was not going to tolerate that. So, we just isolated the teeth we were working on with cotton rolls and our fingers and did a little bit at a time. We were able to get it done, and she handled it very well.

Allowing ample time for the visit, and being sure that the doctor is ready for them when they're ready for the doctor is vitally important. With the little girl who couldn't keep her tongue still, when she came in for her braces, we timed everything else in the clinic so that I would be ready the minute the assistant was ready for her, because that child was not going to sit in the chair and wait for me for even an extra five minutes. I needed to be right there to start applying those braces or we'd have had to start all over. On the other hand, when working with a boy who is severely autistic, we had to put his braces on three brackets at a time because he'd jump out of the chair and run out of the room if we tried to do more. His mother was right there, and helped us calm him down. Thankfully, children usually have a good experience because at the end we praise them and let them know how proud we are of them, and they're always happy about that. It's our goal to make every child feel welcome and appreciated—and that's especially true for these types of patients, because so often people aren't as tolerant or caring as they should be.

GREAT CLINICIANS MAKE ALL THE DIFFERENCE.

Our clinicians are very good at reading a patient's needs and often develop very close relationships with these patients. In fact, usually the patient will ask to see that particular clinician every time they come in. That clinician knows exactly how that patient wants to be treated, what they can tolerate, and what special accommodations need to be made. They're tremendously empathic and great at their jobs, and that's no accident—personality plays a big part in who we hire, in fact, the biggest. You can have someone who's highly skilled and who knows how to do the job, but if they don't have the right personality, then they're not going to be a good fit for our team. We value a great personality in our clinicians because orthodontics is such a people-oriented business.

If you're considering having orthodontics, but you're phobic about dentistry generally or you suffer with claustrophobia, let me reassure you: orthodontics is not a scary ordeal. Yes, there's a little discomfort involved when your teeth start moving, but it's very tolerable. Just focus on what you want to accomplish. Sometimes when we focus on the journey, we think, "Oh, my gosh, that's too hard." But, as with anything in life, if you get stuck on, "How do I get there?" then you'll never accomplish anything. Orthodontics is not going to be a rough road, but it *is* a journey, and it's an easier voyage if you think of it that way. As I tell my adult and teenaged patients, if seven-year-olds can go through this process, so can you.

The anticipation is so much more taxing than the process itself. As one thirteen-year-old said to me after we'd finished putting on her braces, "I was nervous for no reason at all!"

General dentistry patients are sometimes frightened by the noise the dental tools make. I suggest to them that they download a great, calming playlist of their favorite tunes to their phones, tablets, or iPods, invest in a good pair of noise-cancelling headphones, and keep them on during their procedures. I also suggest that if they're fearful of going to the dentist then the best thing they can do is to go every six months, because the more often they go, the less fearful they'll be—and the less likely it is that they'll develop conditions that require more extensive work.

DON'T BE EMBARRASSED—WE'VE SEEN IT ALL!

If it's any comfort, just know that we have seen it all: all kinds of phobias, all kinds of conditions, and all sorts of responses to nervousness. Don't be embarrassed to tell us if you're fearful, because that will help us make you more comfortable. If you need any special accommodations, even if it's just frequent breaks during your procedure, just let us know. No one in any practice should ever, *ever* make you or your child feel self-conscious or unwelcome over these kinds of issues. Everyone's afraid of something in life, after all, and you're entitled to your dignity and our patience. We want all of our patients to tell their general dentists, "I got spoiled at White Brown smiles!"

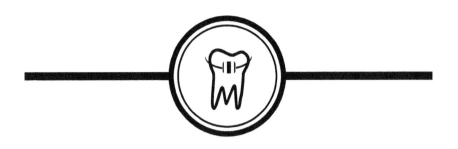

CHAPTER 9

"BUT CAN I AFFORD IT?"

I t's usually not until after the initial smile assessment and consultation is completed (and this is done free of charge at our offices) that we sit down with our patients to talk about the costs and financing for their orthodontic work. It's easy to tell which patients have done research ahead of time on these costs and know what to expect, and those who haven't looked into it and are initially taken aback at the numbers. When we see the "deer in the headlights" look come into their eyes, we explain to them that just because the total bill can be between $3,000 and $6,500, that doesn't mean we expect they pay the entire amount the day the braces goes on. That's when we discuss the options available to them in helping them finance this investment in their or their child's smile.

Some people come in expecting their dental insurance to cover their entire treatment—but usually these plans only cover a portion of the costs, and never one hundred percent. Fortunately, we have options that will help make treatment affordable. We understand that putting down a large sum to get started is difficult for many families, so we've become quite creative in helping parents navigate their alternatives.

One of the ways people access funds to pay for orthodontics is via their flex spending accounts, or the health savings accounts they get through their jobs. Most people don't think of these in terms of dental procedures because they assume they're strictly for medical costs and procedures—but, in fact, they can be used for orthodontics.

Another option for financing is via third-party financing, through companies such as Chase Health Provider, BHG Card, or Care Credit. These third-party financing companies and others like them can help out patients with loans for their orthodontic treatment. Our offices also offer in-house financing, which makes moving forward that much easier for our patients.

Let's discuss these options in greater detail.

GETTING THE MOST OUT OF FLEX SPENDING ACCOUNTS/HEALTH SAVINGS ACCOUNTS

When we work with patients who have flex or health savings accounts, we can help them make it easier on themselves, and avoid flex spending headaches.

The first thing you can do to maximize your potential contribution is to sign up early. For instance, if you know you or your child is going to need orthodontic treatment in the coming year, you should start talking with your Human Resources department early on about enrolling in your employer's flex spending account program so you can maximize that option.

It helps to have some idea of what braces are going to cost, even roughly. Ask, "What is the max I can put in this flex spending account that I can use next year for orthodontic treatment?" Believe it or not, at some companies, you can put anywhere from $2,500 to $5,000 in a flex spending account—and this is before-tax dollars. If this is something your employer offers, it benefits you to get the most into it (and out of it) that you can, because tax-free money goes further when it comes to paying for treatment.

Another thing to be aware of with flex spending accounts is that any change in your status may change your ability to contribute—a death in the family, a marriage or divorce—any personal events can impact and change your status. Even a spouse's loss of job or loss of insurance may allow you to contribute at a higher rate, so be sure to alert your human resources department about status changes and find out how they change your limits.

Please do keep in mind that any money you put into your flex spending account is use it or lose it. If you don't use it during that year it's gone, so it's not a "set it and forget it" kind of a thing. Be aware of the dates within which it must be used, and invest and plan appropriately to reap the maximum tax advantage. At the end of the calendar year, you have up to three months to submit for reimbursement if you have paid for orthodontic treatment or any other medical expense during the previous calendar year. After those three months, you lose whatever is left in that flex spending account. That's why it's important to keep an eye on how much money you anticipate you are going to need, not to put too much in, and to make those status changes if necessary so you have enough but not too much to use during that calendar year.

Luckily, there are several ways to make dental procedures more affordable.

DENTAL INSURANCE

As I mentioned previously, some people come in assuming their dental insurance will cover half of their orthodontic costs because of the language of their policy. But you need to look carefully to understand the language—it's 50 percent of a *lifetime max*, not 50 percent of the cost of whatever the procedure or treatment is.

What we find is that on average, most dental insurance policies will pay anywhere from $1,000 to about $2,500 toward orthodontic treatment. There are some insurance policies that pay more than that, but they're few and far between. That means the average person is looking at $1,000 toward an orthodontic bill of about $6,500. If your insurance tells you they'll pay 50 percent of a lifetime max of $2,000, then you know the insurance benefit is $1,000. When patients come in with their dental insurance, we'll review it with them and help them understand the often-confusing jargon so they're able to best take advantage of what their policy provides.

THIRD-PARTY FINANCING

An option many patients like is going through a company that offers third-party financing. There's always an interest charge for a period beyond six months, as with nearly any loan, and the length of the term you choose and the amount of money you borrow determines that rate. Say you go with a company like Care Credit, one of these loan providers, and you take out a loan of $1,000 for one year. You may pay a relatively minimal interest rate on that $1,000 because it's a year-long term. You can extend that to two years, but your interest cost is going to be higher. These contracts can be confusing, so we always take the time to go over the fine print and costs with patients so they can make the best decision. Not everyone can come up with the down payment they need to start treatment out of pocket, and sometimes patients like this kind of financing because they can take a $1,000 loan out and put that toward their down payment, and then pay this third party back over time at the agreed-upon rate.

Sometimes we have a patient whose insurance covers $1,000, and they have a health savings account for that year with another $2,000. That patient will sometimes use third-party financing to cover the entire remaining balance so they don't owe the practice anything. That works for some people because they don't want to feel like, "I have to make sure I pay my orthodontic bill," or, "I need to make sure my child is being taken care of." Now that their commitment to the office is paid in full, they're only dealing with their lender in terms of payments.

IN-HOUSE FINANCING

We find that most patients and parents find in-house financing is the best way to go, particularly in our office because we don't charge an interest rate but they still get to pay us over time. Depending on the patient's circumstances, they pay whatever down payment they've agreed to make, and then the balance is paid off in monthly installments. We ask the responsible party to put this on a direct payment basis (autodraft) so that money is paid on a fixed schedule directly from their bank account or via their credit card. Patients like this option because it's something they don't have to think about. They've set an amount they're comfortable with and it's being automatically drafted from their accounts. We work with them to make sure that the monthly payment is affordable for them, and patients really appreciate the convenience (and lack of interest payments!).

Of course, there are people who are simply uncomfortable taking out any kind of loan or paying over time for treatment. They generally come in having saved up the entire amount necessary for treatment, because they knew it would be needed and they've planned and saved ahead. These patients get a special break because, in most practices, there is an additional 5 to 10 percent discount on treatment that's paid for in full. Why? Because now our staff doesn't have to keep track of your account, so the practice saves money as well.

WE'LL WORK WITH YOU.

We once had a patient who was extremely worried about finances: "I know this is something my child needs. But how am I going to be able to afford this?" he asked. We ended up setting up payments for the entire amount, even the down payment. Because he couldn't come up with the initial $1,000 we worked it out so that he was able to pay $250 for four consecutive months and then started his regular monthly payment, which was about $180. That made it affordable and enabled him to get his child the treatment he knew she needed. We were happy to help. On another occasion, where the patient told us, "$200 is a bit much for me," we allowed him to extend his monthly payment and had him on automatic draft so we didn't have to monitor whether or not his payments were being made. This allowed him to get started in treatment without any financial problems.

Our goal is to help patients however we can to be able to afford orthodontic treatment. We're more than willing to get creative in financing, as long as it makes sense for the practice, and the patient can handle it—we'll find an option or a combination of options to make it work.

Another patient was worried about making monthly payments—but she had maximized her health savings accounts, so every year we put that lump sum toward her bill, about $1,500 per year. Instead of having her put up that entire $1,500 as a down payment, we put it on her account and let it bill out, because she couldn't afford to make the monthly payments beyond what she contributed to her health savings account. That meant we could stretch that payment toward the next eleven months of the year, when she got another lump sum from the health savings account. We did that until her account was paid out in full.

I realize not every practice is as flexible in this regard as we are. You still sometimes come across those offices that say, "Okay, your bill is $6,500. We want 25 percent down now." While there is a segment of society for which coming up with that kind of money isn't an issue, others just can't manage to pay so much at once with all the other obligations they have already. They search out practices like ours who are willing to work with them and create options they can live with. We've helped literally thousands of people through this process afford orthodontic treatment for themselves or their child.

COSTS VERSUS VALUE? NO CONTEST!

When you're weighing the costs and payments, remember—this isn't just a beauty treatment. I realize that when you initially consider the costs of orthodontics, you may well feel, "Oh, my gosh, this is a burden." However, when you look at orthodontic treatment and the psychological effect it can have on a person for the rest of their lives—on their ability to move forward positively and successfully in life—you begin to see the costs for what they really represent: a critical investment in you or your child's future. The question then is no longer, "How can I afford this?" but rather, "How can I afford not to?"

People spend money on all kinds things that don't last—people will take their children to Disney World, or buy a new car. There are a million things people spend money on that aren't nearly as impactful as orthodontics. That car loses significant value the minute you drive it off the lot, but as long as you keep your teeth, you'll reap the benefits of orthodontics. This investment will just keep paying dividends.

We had a dad who brought his child in because he wanted to get her started with braces, but when he heard the costs he just couldn't see how he could afford it. The treatment coordinator could see the disappointment in his face—he wanted it so much for his child—and she told him, "Okay. We can do this. What are you capable of paying monthly?" They talked about the monthly payments he was making already—the average person pays $200 for a monthly cable bill for instance—so that when it's broken down to those terms it's easier to see it's doable. The treatment coordinator was able to put this father at ease. He was ecstatic to be able to say, "Okay. Let's get my daughter started."

One mother said to me, "This is the only investment I can make that I don't lose my money on; it's an investment in my child and in my child's future." A beautiful smile is a gift that lasts a lifetime, and keeps paying dividends.

HELP FOR THE NEEDIEST

Of course, there are cases where people simply cannot pay—no matter what the financing options are—and there is help for them, too. In some cases where there is extreme need, and a child's health is endangered by debilitating issues, we've reduced our fees. Here in South Carolina, The Children Rehabilitative Services will pay for orthodontic treatment for the most severe cases—not every practice accepts these patients, but my practice certainly does. We aren't compensated at our normal rate for orthodontic treatment, however, we absorb the loss. We view this as our contribution to the people of our community. I am extremely passionate about giving back to our community. We probably treat five to ten new cases per month at reduced fees through Medicaid and Children's Rehabilitative Services.

One little girl of about twelve came in with a really extreme protrusion of her front teeth. She really needed help, and I could tell she was getting teased—my heart went out to her. She didn't smile; she barely talked. Her bite was really bad, but I knew braces could fix her bite without the need for surgery, though it would require some extractions. She had severe overbite and overjet with lots of crowding; her front teeth were basically sticking straight out of her face. That's how bad it was.

After her exam, she and her mother met with our treatment coordinator to talk about payment options. After they left the office, I asked the treatment coordinator, "Okay, how did that go? When is she going to get started?"

She told me, "Mom can't afford this. She has no means to pay for braces." None of the options we put out there would work for her because of her financial situation. That wasn't acceptable to me. I said, "We have to help this child." So, we filled out the Children's

Rehabilitative Services paperwork for her. I led that effort because I knew that if this child didn't get help, her life was going to be miserable. It crushed my heart to see her when she walked in—and I wasn't going to let her go through life that way.

She got approved, and we began treatment. Now when she comes in and I talk to her she's still very timid, but I can see that she feels better about herself because she smiles now, and looks at you when you speak to her. There are probably some other issues that need to be worked out as far as her self-esteem is concerned, but orthodontics has helped tremendously. She's in retainers now, and nearly done with the retention portion of her treatment. I know it's been a life-changing event for her—and her mother.

I'm happy to also work with Smiles Change Lives, the nonprofit that puts me and other orthodontists together with children who can't afford the orthodontic work they desperately need. We do it pro bono, and it's a great, great feeling to know I'm giving back. This helps out those low-income children whose cases aren't so extreme that they qualify for the Children's Rehabilitative Services program, but whose appearances can and will negatively impact them socially and emotionally. Those are patients we're happy to jump in and help. To date, my offices have donated more than $250,000 in services.

Smiles really *do* change lives. In the next chapter, I'll share some of my favorite stories of patients whose lives were changed dramatically for the better by orthodontic treatment.

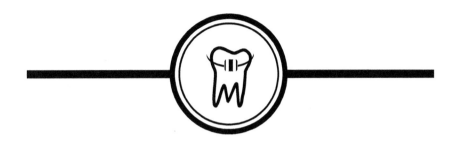

CHAPTER 10

"YOU CHANGED MY LIFE!"

SHE'S A SWEETHEART, BUT HER TEETH . . .

"Honey, there's a little girl at church who really needs your help." As usual, my husband, a deacon at our church, had stayed behind after services to chat with other parishioners as I scurried out of church, trying to get our two restive little boys home to get them fed. He returned home to tell me about this little girl, Holly—bursting with warmth and personality, and as sweet as she could be—but with teeth that were about as bad as *they* could be.

"I was talking to her and all I could see was teeth everywhere," he said. "You have to get her in the office; I couldn't believe what I was looking at. You've got to help her."

Now, parishioners often approach him to ask about my services, and his response is usually, "That's my wife. Talk to her." But Holly's plight was something he'd really taken to heart—it was as though in interceding for her, he was asking for a personal favor. He kept repeating, "There are teeth everywhere."

We spoke to her grandparents the next Sunday, and I told them, "Okay. We'd like to help. Let's get her in. Let's assess and see what's going on and what needs to happen from there."

The day Holly came in the office, my staff had the same reaction as my husband. When they took her x-rays, the x-ray technician said, "Dr. White Brown, you've got to come see this." They wanted me to look at it privately. "Oh, my God. We've never seen anything like this before," the technician kept saying. She had worked in the industry for twenty-plus years, so I knew the x-rays had to be pretty alarming.

And they were right—I was astonished by what I saw. Holly had so many extra teeth! I had never seen anything like it before. It's not unusual to run into a patient with an extra tooth or two—three was the most I'd ever come across previously—but Holly had about fourteen too many. Her teeth were (unsurprisingly) crowded—and x-rays showed that a lot of these extra teeth hadn't even fully come in yet. I was happy that she got to me when she did; she really did need help, and fast.

After her exam, I sat down with her mother: "This is going to be a very involved treatment. We're going to have to get other practitioners involved, like the oral surgeon and a general dentist, to help us with her case." We got started.

This case took nearly four years to finish, and Holly was so grateful when we were done; she just couldn't stop hugging me. Her parents and family were grateful too, because even though she'd always had such a bright, lit-up personality, she lit up even more now that she was proud of her smile. It was a great success, and we were elated our practice could do that for her and her family. Holly needed a smile as beautiful as her personality, and now she had one. Without a doubt, the best thing about being an orthodontist is that the results we achieve are so often hugely dramatic in the effect they have on a patient's appearance and self-esteem. It's wonderfully gratifying to hear, "You changed my life!" and I love that I get to hear it so often.

I NEVER THOUGHT THIS DAY WOULD COME!

When twenty-eight-year-old Gina came to us for her initial consultation, I could see that her case was severe. She had a such large open bite—as a child she had been a thumb sucker—that when she opened her mouth, you could not see any teeth on top at all. Actually, you couldn't see any teeth on the bottom either, because her open bite was that large. The lower front teeth were intruded—in other words, they were submerged in the gums because of the thumb sucking. The upper teeth were up so high and out that when she talked all you could see was her tongue. Most orthodontists would look at that and say, "You definitely need jaw surgery to correct this." But because she couldn't afford it, and because she had a lot of other dental work that needed to be done, I agreed to do everything I could to help.

We started off with braces on the upper and lower teeth to start unraveling the crowding. She did have to have some teeth removed, and because we periodically had to remove wires and brackets so she could have dental work performed her case moved slowly. We did it this way because there was so much crowding that it made it difficult for the dentist to adequately perform good restorations that wouldn't have to be replaced after orthodontics. She was patient, and we moved her treatment along slowly but surely.

We were able to fix her bite and improve her appearance far beyond what she'd ever dared to hope for, giving her the beautiful smile she'd always dreamed of. The day her braces came off, Gina wept tears of joy. She told us, "I never thought this day would come!" I'm so glad she found the courage to come in for that initial consultation when others had told her that her case was hopeless without surgery, and that we were able to help her.

I DON'T WANT MY DAUGHTER TO SUFFER AS I DID.

Sometimes it takes seeing the results of orthodontics on someone else to make a person realize how much having a beautiful smile would mean to them, and to give them the courage to go for it themselves. Barbara brought her daughter Michelle into us for an initial consultation because she herself had suffered through having terrible teeth her whole life, and was determined to make sure her little girl didn't have to go through that. Like the patient I discussed previously, she'd been told several times over the years by different practitioners that her case demanded surgery, and that without it her bite and her smile couldn't be corrected. As I talked with Barbara, I couldn't help but notice that her issues were very similar to what I'd seen in her daughter's mouth. When I told her, "Yes, we can help Michelle," the relief that washed over her face was something to see—she teared up as she thanked me. Sparing her little girl the pain and humiliation she'd experienced was hugely important to her, and knowing this was possible without surgery was a great relief. When our treatment coordinator sat down with Barbara they were able to work out a payment plan that put Michelle's treatment well within her reach.

When Michelle was through with her treatment, she was transformed. Her smile was gorgeous and her mom was overjoyed. That was when she asked me if I could take a look at her mouth and possibly treat her, too. I'd been hoping she would ask! We got her into braces, and now both mother and daughter have matching, beautiful smiles. Barbara admitted that she'd been afraid it was too late for her, but it's never too late to make an improvement in the way you feel about yourself.

YOU'RE NEVER TOO OLD TO IMPROVE YOUR SMILE.

An older gentleman in his seventies who came in to see me. He had an upper denture that was due to be replaced, so we began the process of putting his natural lower teeth into better alignment. That way when he got his upper denture redone his teeth will fit together much better than they did before. And yes, he was excited at the prospect of having a great smile—so clearly, you're never too old to care about how you look!

THANK YOU FOR HELPING ME LOOK PRETTY ON MY WEDDING DAY!

Sometimes it takes a big occasion to make a person decide to pursue orthodontic treatment. I'm treating Gloria, a soon-to-be bride, right now. We started working with her about eight months ago when her fiancé popped the question. We're aligning her teeth as quickly as we

"A STRONG, POSITIVE SELF-IMAGE IS THE BEST POSSIBLE PREPARATION FOR SUCCESS IN LIFE."

—DR. JOYCE BROTHERS

can, and she hasn't got much further to go. More than anything she wanted a beautiful smile on her wedding day, and she got it—two weeks ago we took her braces off for her wedding day. Gloria got married, had her photographs done, and earlier this week we put her braces back on so we can begin to complete her treatment. She was so proud to show me her wedding photos: "Thank you for making me look so pretty," she told me.

I get a lot of brides-to-be who decide there will never be a better occasion to look their best—and they're right. The difference between dieting, or makeup and hair, or finding the perfect dress, and their smile is, of course, that they'll have their beautiful smiles for the rest of their lives. Sometimes if they come in early enough we're able to complete their treatment entirely before their wedding portraits and their wedding. But other times we may have to start, stop for a little while, and then proceed with treatment when they're done.

WE CHANGE MORE THAN SMILES.

Sometimes I change lives in ways that go far beyond creating a beautiful smile, and that was certainly the case with Carmen, a fifteen-year-old girl who came to see us for a consultation. Part of the initial consultation process is taking a full set of x-rays. This allows us to see the underlying structure of the mouth, and helps us spot any pathologies under the gums or in the bones that we wouldn't be able to see otherwise. Typically, we take a panoramic x-ray and a cephalometric x-ray, as well.

Looking at her x-rays, I saw immediately that while one of her nostrils was completely normal and clear, the other one was totally obstructed. It was clogged, which seemed unusual. While she was in the chair, I held one nostril closed, and said, "Okay, breathe in."

She was able to do that. Then I switched nostrils and said, "Breathe in again, please," and she couldn't take in even the tiniest bit of air. I turned to her mother, "Mom, you need to take her to the ENT. There's definitely an obstruction there." Her mother was astonished; clearly the obstruction had been there so long that Carmen wasn't even aware that it was abnormal. She'd probably never even mentioned it to her mother, who I guess must have been thinking, "Oh, it's probably just a stuffy nose or allergies."

But when the ENT spotted the same obstruction when he examined her, and she had to have minor surgery to remove it. Carmen was amazed at the difference that removing the obstruction had made, because she began breathing so much better. It really changed her quality of life—certainly in a way she hadn't anticipated—when she came to the orthodontist to fix her smile!

SMILES CHANGE LIVES—AND WE CHANGE SMILES.

The patients I see through the charity Smiles Change Lives are among the most amazed by and grateful for the results we give them. I remember one family in particular who brought in Luke, a twelve-year-old boy. His grandparents were his primary caregivers and lived on a fixed income, so without financial assistance they wouldn't have been able to afford the braces Luke desperately needed. He came in for the consultation, and I made my recommendations. At my suggestion, they went through the application process with Smiles Change Lives, and when his application was accepted we brought Luke on as a patient. His grandparents were overwhelmed when they heard he'd be treated in our offices for free and couldn't stop thanking me.

We put his braces on that day and I was moving on to the next patient when my office manager came and got me—Luke's whole family was in the waiting room wanting to meet me. When I walked in, they were all beaming with joy. Grandma gave me a big hug and told me how grateful and how amazed the entire family was that we were donating this service and devoting our time to her grandson, because otherwise they knew that they wouldn't have been able to afford braces for him. Of course, every parent or grandparent wants the best for their child. The entire family was shaking my hand, hugging me, blessing me. I felt so humbled, and so thankful I was able to be of service and give to this family something that felt impossible to them prior to accepting him into my practice. Being able to serve Luke gave me more pleasure than it did the family. I was overwhelmed by their gratitude.

I'm so passionate about what I do—and about the Smiles Change Lives foundation—because, as a child, I remember the dentist telling my mom that I needed braces. I remember my mother telling me afterward that we couldn't afford it. Thankfully, my teeth were not the worst, but I grew up knowing that I wanted to have them fixed. My mom and dad had eight children, and the family budget just couldn't stretch to accommodate orthodontics. It wasn't until I was an adult that I was able to get the braces I'd always wanted, and the smile I'd dreamed of. That makes this work especially meaningful for me, because I know what it feels like to long for a beautiful smile your parents can't afford to give you. I know what it's like to have your self-esteem bruised by the things your peers (and sometimes even adults) say about your appearance, and it gives me great satisfaction to give other children what I had to wait until adulthood to acquire.

NOBODY CAN KNOW I'M WEARING BRACES.

Sometimes patients come to me with challenges that are made all the more difficult by their special requirements. One patient who stands out in my memory was Aaron, a nice young man of about thirty. I had treated his wife previously, who'd sent him in to see what we could do for him. He had very nice teeth, but they were terribly crowded and there just wasn't enough room in his mouth for them all.

After his exam, we sat down to talk. Aaron was adamant that if we were going to correct his smile that it had to be with Invisalign because he didn't want anyone to know he was wearing braces. He was a realtor, and he told me, "I'm always talking to people. I don't want braces in my mouth."

I tried to talk him out of it. I told him, "You're going to have to have extractions. There's too much crowding here. We cannot do this with Invisalign alone."

But Aaron wasn't about to be talked out of his choice, or talked into any extractions: "No. If we're going to do this, it's going to be Invisalign, period," he told me.

I thought a moment, then I said, "Okay. Well, we'll try. We'll see how far we get, and how much we can get accomplished."

Sixty Invisalign trays later, he had the smile he wanted. It took him an awfully long time, and there were multiple revisions and additional trays had to be fabricated for him, but we were able to get him the results he wanted, the way he wanted. I remember at one point getting one box of thirty trays and having to resubmit for additional trays. But we just kept going.

We had to create little spaces here and there throughout treatment, but we were able to correct his smile. Again, it took over three years, but today Aaron has the most gorgeous smile ever. It helped that he started out with big, beautiful teeth, but now that they're well-aligned his smile is awesome. And we did it all with Invisalign. He was thrilled with the outcome.

IS MY CASE HOPELESS?

So many people come to us having been told that they need surgery, or having been told by multiple orthodontists that their cases can't be treated. Sometimes these folks gave up searching for help years ago. But there are so many new technologies available to us that weren't there before, so we're able to do a lot more than we used to. And while it takes a lot more work on the orthodontist's part, we're also able to do a lot more than used to be possible without surgery—for instance, treatment that we couldn't perform before the advent of Temporary Anchorage Devices (TADs), and other similar technology, especially in adult patients who have several missing teeth.

Before this technology became available, we would have had to tell them, "I'm sorry. We can't do this, because you don't have any back teeth, so we don't have any anchors." Now we have anchors that we can place there to help move these teeth. Again, it may take longer without surgery, but now it's possible that these problems can be corrected without it.

The fact is, in dentistry in general we don't want to do a lot of the extractions that we might have done in the past, and that's partly because of issues it can create around sleep apnea, a serious sleep disorder in which an obstructed airway causes a person to repeatedly stop breathing during sleep, sometimes hundreds of times in a night. Sleep apnea can cause a whole array of other health problems, and it's not something to take lightly.

When we take out teeth and move teeth back, we're effectively shoving the patient's tonsils into the back of their mouth. If a patient already has issues with sleep apnea, we can make that situation worse when we take out teeth. Now don't get me wrong, there are instances that warrant taking out teeth when there's just no other possible way, but what we're doing more often now in the industry is saying, "Let's just figure out how we can correct this problem without taking out teeth and complicating a breathing problem," because you certainly want to be able to breathe, and we don't want to create a new problem in the process of solving an existing one. Now we look at every case to see how we can treat it without having to perform extractions.

PARENTS KNOW BEST.

Sometimes it takes a determined parent to help a child over their resistance to getting braces; the parent knows what a difference it will make once it's done, even if the child can't see that far ahead. Thirteen-year-old Gayla was an unwilling patient whose mother told me, "I know she doesn't want this, but I know what she needs and I'm the parent, so we're going to make this happen." Gayla was not a happy camper. It was evident in her body language and her overall attitude that she had zero interest in being there. If she spoke at all, it was in answer to a question—and usually just a word or two. Typically, we create relationships with our patients because we see them so often. We talk to them a lot. It's a very personal relationship because you're up close to the person, and you're in their mouth. That usually sparks some conversation about life and whatever else is going on in their world.

With Gayla though, in the beginning we got nothing but attitude. When she was asked to do something as simple as turning her head or opening her mouth she would do it reluctantly, and with a lot of eye rolling.

But once we got her started and her results were beginning to show, she loved the fact that her teeth and her bite were changing for the better, and she actually became one of our best and most compliant patients. She became far more cooperative, and much nicer than she had been in the beginning. When we were done and she had a beautiful smile, she came to me and thanked me—"I know I didn't want this done, but I'm so glad my mom made me go through with it. Thank you for being so patient!"

THE GIRL WHO HID HER SMILE

Looking back, one of my first cases was also one of the most satisfying: sixteen-year-old Callie, who, unlike Gayla, was eager to get her teeth fixed. Her mouth was terribly crowded, and she hated her teeth; she was always covering up her smile, and turning away or laughing behind her hand. Hers was one of those cases where the canines were sitting under her lip because there was no room for them in the arch. It was uncomfortable when she ate because every time she moved her lip, that tooth irritated her lip.

When we were done, Callie was so happy that she was smiling all the time. I was nearly as thrilled by her transformation as she was, and I asked her if I could use her photo in my advertising. She was delighted at the thought of being my model, and agreed enthusiastically.

That gesture of covering up the smile is one I see often, and it always breaks my heart a little bit. How sad it is that a natural expression that expresses your joy to those around you is so ugly to you that you habitually hide it. Those habits take years to make; a lot of suffering must have gone into forming them!

You can see why I love my work. It's not everyone who gets a chance to change lives for the better, and I'm grateful every day that I am afforded this opportunity.

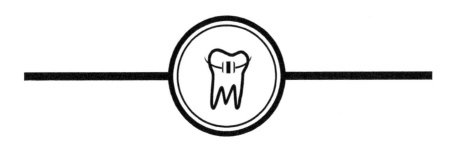

IN CLOSING

O rthodontics can change someone's life. Those who don't understand how challenging it is for someone to be ashamed of their smile tend to shrug it off—what's the big deal about having crooked teeth? But twenty years in practice have opened my eyes to the far-reaching emotional impact an ugly smile can have. The other day a grandmother brought her granddaughter to see me; she was being picked on in school because of her awful looking teeth, and Grandma had had enough: "Whatever I have to do, I want her to be happy about her smile," she told me. Grandma had been bullied herself as a girl, and knew the pain it was causing her granddaughter. These emotions run deep, and given the proven impact a person's appearance has on their confidence and on their potential earnings throughout their life, it's certainly more than a superficial issue.

I hope that if you're contemplating orthodontics for your child or for yourself, this book has answered any questions you might have had, and shown you how easy it is to get the smile you've always dreamed of. Advances in orthodontic technology have made treatment easier and faster than was possible before, and it's more affordable than you probably think—not to mention the initial smile assessment is free. If you'd like to know more, check out my website—whitebrownsmiles.com—or give us a call and come on in. I'm all about changing the world one smile at a time, and I'd love to help you uncover the beautiful smile you've always wanted.

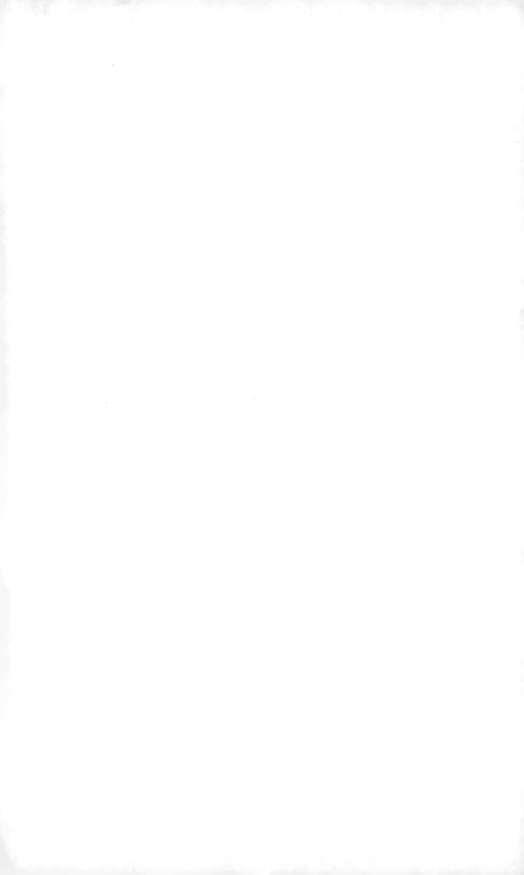

GO THE EXTRA MILE
INVEST IN YOUR SMILE.

A smile says a lot about a person—even how confident you are in pursuing your dreams. Exactly what does your smile say about you?

If you've been putting off making the smile of your dreams a reality because of finances, fear, or lack of faith, brace yourself: Dr. Kerry White Brown is here to tell you that your dreams may be more in reach than you thought. A winning smile can change your or your child's life—all it takes is this book to find out how.

In *A Lifetime of Sensational Smiles*, Dr. White Brown explains orthodontics in a simplistic way to relieve all of your fears and show you why your smile is something worth investing in.

So if the thought of going to the orthodontist or dentist has you grinding your teeth with anxiety, Dr. White Brown will put your mind at ease in this refreshing read about the importance of pursuing orthodontics to help you achieve your very own Sensational Smile.

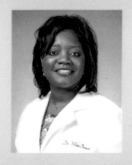

DR. KERRY WHITE BROWN

is a practicing orthodontist in Columbia, South Carolina. With a specialty degree in orthodontics from Howard University College of Dentistry, Dr. White Brown has made it her mission to give each and every one of her patients the optimal care they deserve on their journey to their unique Sensational Smile.

Advantage®

advantagefamily.com

ISBN 978-1-59932-803-4

90000

9 781599 328034

TENKO!

RANGOON JAIL

**THE AMAZING STORY OF SGT. JOHN
BOYD'S SURVIVAL AS A POW IN A
NOTORIOUS JAPANESE PRISON CAMP**

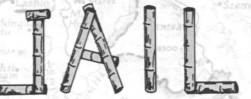

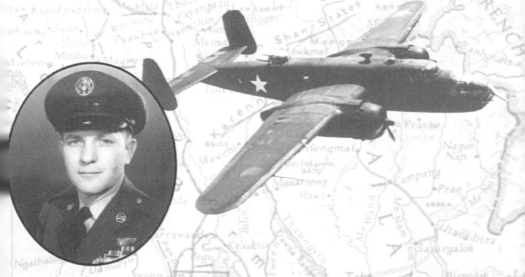

by JOHN BOYD *with* GARY GARTH